Religion and Medicine

Also published by SCM Press

A Sociological Yearbook of Religion in Britain
edited by David Martin

A Sociological Yearbook of Religion in Britain · 2
edited by David Martin

Religion and Medicine

A Discussion

Edited by M. A. H. Melinsky

Published for the Institute of
Religion and Medicine by

SCM PRESS LTD

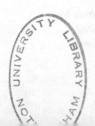

334 00673 2

First published 1970
by SCM Press Ltd
56 Bloomsbury Street London WC1

© *SCM Press Ltd 1970*

Printed in Great Britain by
Billing & Sons Limited
Guildford and London

CONTENTS

CONTENTS

PREFACE

At one time religion and medicine, priest and doctor shared a common concern and exercised a common ministry. We may, for instance, recall some of the injunctions – both priestly and medical – contained in the book *Leviticus* or the Christian provision of hospitals. Salvation and healing were but different ways of being made whole, though it was never correct to regard the two concepts as synonymous. Then, in the seventeenth century, came the great divide. Each ministry started its independent journey and took its sailing orders from a conceptual mapping which has the Cartesian mind-body dichotomy at its centre, though it is only fair to Descartes to recall that he had himself more *arrières pensées* than he has subsequently been given credit for.

From the side of medicine at any rate, Descartes was regarded as a godsend. F. G. Garrison, writing his monumental *History of Medicine*, which contains a full and detailed account of medical development ranging from primitive and prehistoric times to the scientific medicine of some forty years ago, argues that 'medicine could not begin to be medicine until it was disassociated from magic and religion'. It was, claims Garrison, necessary for medical development that the functions of priest, magician and medicine man – the same person in primitive society – should 'become specialized and differentiated'.

When there was this explicit division of labour, it seemed as if any clergyman or doctor who supposed he had something to offer of direct relevance to the other, was bound to be either superstitious or a crank. Garrison himself remarks ruefully that 'even today medicine sometimes partakes of magical and mystical (religious) as well as of scientific elements'.

But the broadening of the spectrum of illness; the knowledge that we now have of the complex inter-relationship there can be between psychological and biological factors in health and sickness; the growing awareness that the ministry of healing is inevitably a matter of teamwork – this following not only from specialist developments within medicine itself, and from the technological developments relating to medical skills and apparatus, but also from the development of social medicine; the notion of a therapeutic community whose boundaries cannot be restricted to the hospital curtilage – all these point to the need for novel and important bridge-building between the two disciplines.

The Institute of Religion and Medicine was founded precisely to make possible frontier work between the two professions and disciplines, to allow doctors and clergy to meet and grapple with common problems. It is in this kind of context that the papers produced in this book arose.

Has medicine concentrated on disease to the neglect of the person who is ill? Has it been disease-attacking rather than health-enhancing? How far can 'repentance' be interpreted as the 'working through of anxiety'? What insights into human nature can be derived from studying the conflicts and anxieties of those who are sick? How far does the therapeutic community, by raising issues relating to anxiety and authority, provide us with helpful ideas for our understanding of any community? How does a community – church or hospital – discover a structure which better expresses its purpose, and how do we succeed in getting an understanding of that purpose right down the line and throughout the community? What is involved from the point of priest and doctor, in communicating news, be that news the gospel or news of some terminal illness? Both doctors and clergy cannot but gain from Dr Saunders' chapter on 'Dimensions of Death' written, as she always writes, with a detailed practical knowledge as well as with deep insight and sensitivity. In these ways the essays help us to elucidate for both doctors and clergy what Canon Sydney Evans rightly speaks of as the distinctiveness and yet the inter-relation of their respective ministries to the needs of humanity.

The essays also introduce us to the possibilities and difficulties of training in pastoral care, whether under the auspices of clinical theology or as developed in the USA. How far, asks Dr Lambourne, is the unsatisfactoriness of many American schemes the result of 'conceptual deficiencies which stem in their turn from the absence of tough dialogue between medicine and theology'? Here, however, is a book calculated to encourage a tough dialogue between medicine and theology and one that comes from sharing common problems and bringing to those problems the specialities of different disciplines, which can nevertheless be used together in the service of the person who is the concern of them all.

IAN DUNELM:

1 Our Growth as Persons

Sydney Evans

Canon Sydney Evans was elected President of the Institute of Religion and Medicine for 1968-1969, the fifth in its history. He has been actively associated with the Institute since its foundation.

As Dean of King's College, London, Canon Evans is much concerned with the preparation of men for the ordained ministry of the Church of England, not least for their training in pastoral care.

This chapter is based on a talk given to the 1968 Annual Meeting of the Guild of Saint Raphael. It was originally printed, as spoken, in *Chrism*, the Guild's quarterly magazine, and is here reproduced in slightly modified form by kind permission of the Editor.

Christianity is concerned with our growth as persons. This growth is determined by certain physical and biological necessities which it is the task of science to explore, and by an individual's reaction to those necessities in the light of perceived possibilities which it is the task of education, of psychotherapy, of religion to explore. Understanding human nature has become even more complex and fascinating today than it has been found to be in the past, and of its fascination in the past art and literature are evidence enough. When we (as individuals) have time off from the business of life to reflect, our deepest questions are normally – Who am I? What may I hope? What should I do?

Just as the shape of a full-grown tree indicates by the curious configuration of branches that growth takes place in relation both to inherent characteristics and energies and also to external forces and pressures, so too human emotional growth and development happens in relation to various necessities and perceptions. Heredity and environment, nature and nurture are familiar antitheses which modern knowledge spells out in terms of genetic inheritance and DNA, as well as in terms of social conditioning in the context of family, neighbourhood, school, church.

Christian faith speaks of the need for persons to discover their highest possibilities of personalness by relating to Jesus the Christ as he is presented in the bible, in the living tradition of thought and worship in the Christian community, in the personal lives of those who have been open to his influence. But this Christian understanding of the high possibilities of personalness open to every man and woman – this Christian talk about 'spirituality' – needs in these days to be well and truly rooted and grounded in that understanding of human nature which is all the time being advanced by those whose study is the medical and human sciences. It may therefore not be unhelpful to explore a little that process of understanding which we call diagnosis as part of our desire as doctors and clergy to see better what are our individual roles in their distinctiveness and in their inter-relation. The unitive centre of our professions is the human person as he is and as he is capable of becoming – physically, mentally, emotionally, spiritually. Health, as understood by the doctor and psychotherapist, and salvation as understood by the Christian community, are neither identical nor wholly unrelated.

In the work of healing and of salvation diagnosis, genuine understanding of the way things are really, is of supreme importance. The priest as consultant and the general practitioner as consultant and the psychiatrist as consultant are equally concerned to analyse the symptoms that are presented and to discover as far as possible what are the underlying causes of those symptoms. This is as necessary for the priest who is being consulted by a person in difficulties about faith and prayer as it is for the psychiatrist who is being consulted by a person who cannot cope with some situation or relationship. Diagnosis is a demanding duty. It requires time, and time is not adequately available for the busy GP. It requires patience, a capacity for patient listening and analysis which needs to be sustained by an inner conviction sufficient to counterbalance whatever personal antipathies the consultant may feel – not least his own weariness. It requires skill, partly to be learned but partly to be achieved by the development of empathy as a result of spending time in listening over a number of years. It requires also, I suspect, an element of that sensitivity we call intuition because we do not know what it is but recognize that there is something for which the word intuition stands: it would seem to be both a personal gift and also the result of experience of the kind I referred to above as growing out of empathy. I expect that the difference between one diagnostician and another is not necessarily the fact that they have had a different training but that they have both had similar training and one has this 'flair', this ability to consider two pieces of information in juxtaposition and to find himself led on to think of a third – the underlying cause of the symptoms.

In terms of the experience of the general practitioner, the pressure on him or her of the number of patients waiting in the waiting-room must sometimes result in a diagnosis that is superficial or inadequate, if not actually wrong. The patient cannot articulate what he is really feeling. The doctor takes the short cut and writes out a prescription for a drug. For this reason if for no other the Royal Commission on Medical Education, the Todd Report, is to be welcomed. With more GPs and more adequately trained GPs we may hope that there will be a gain in the time and the skill available for more adequate diagnosis.

But whatever diagnosis anyone makes, it will always be provisional. It will only be the best a person can do with the information presented, and may have to be revised in the light of more information. Initial symptoms, in the clinic and in the confessional, may suggest a number of different possible causes: only more careful analysis can narrow down the possibility so that the actual disease can be more accurately diagnosed.

In our technologically advancing society we can expect that the pressure of need of sick people for diagnosis and treatment will result in more mechanical methods of gathering information. It is already possible for a new patient presenting himself to have a blood sample taken and for this blood sample to be rapidly analysed by a computer-controlled process so that the doctor seeing the new patient already has in front of him a considerable amount of accurate information before he begins to talk with the patient himself. The use of modern procedures to aid diagnosis is likely to change the pattern of medical practice increasingly: one of the most interesting chapters in the Todd Report is that which speaks of the *future* of the medical services.

One of the main developments in this area of diagnosis – this attempt to discover what it really is that is inhibiting this person from fulfilling his role in life (which is at least in part what we mean when we talk of illness) – one of the main developments in recent years is indicated by the word 'psychosomatic'. It is interesting

that a word had to be invented in order to draw attention to the
fact that the emotional state of a person can affect his physical state
and vice versa. In other words a human person has to be considered
as a totality, and physical complaints may well have aggravating
causes which arise from aspects of personal experience which we
may call emotional, psychological or sociological. A GP in these
days can no longer treat the body as a separable organism – as if
a patient takes his body to the garage and the garage mechanic
does whatever he thinks is required to put the machine on to the
road again. A GP who is moving in his understanding within the
world of today rather than of yesterday will know that a patient is a
person whose biological and psychological and sociological history
have to be taken into account in arriving at a diagnosis.

Many a GP in a quiet hour, when he can be persuaded to relax
and talk over his work, will say that a high proportion of the people
who come to him do not really need drugs; they need someone who
has the time and understanding to listen to what is really causing
them to feel depressed and unable to cope. What is really worrying
them is not lethargy and lassitude of body but the fact that life is
difficult, pressures are heavy, people are needling them, or they
are themselves anxious and afraid. Psychosomatic awareness is
one of the most important developments in diagnosis: perhaps
it will soon be possible to abandon this word because what it was
invented to emphasize has become a normal element in the diagnostician's approach.

The evidence suggests that in our modern society the number of
people who in one way or another need help for emotional stress or
mental illness is increasing. But for all our advances in knowledge
we seem still to be only at the beginning of procedures for accurate
diagnosis. The more we know the more tentative do we become.
A continuing debate appears to be ahead of us between those who in
emotional illness adhere to therapy by analysis and those who
adhere to therapy by drugs. There are biochemists who deny the
reality of psychological illness: emotional and mental stress they
say are chemically based: what is needed is more accurate knowledge of biochemistry and pharmacology. There are many psychiatrists who, while welcoming and using the drugs made available by
pharmacology, would say that mental illness cannot be cured by
pharmacology alone: there is need for speech between patient and
doctor, the attempt to enable the patient to discover and articulate

his own personal experiences which underlie his present condition. There are again many psychoanalysts who would claim that the root causes of certain conditions of mental illness are historically based in experiences and relationships of childhood which need to be uncovered and re-lived in order that the patient may be set free from the tyranny of repressed childhood feelings of hate and guilt. And there are some who use drugs such as LSD in order to speed up the process of remembering so that the root causes of the present distress can be more rapidly reached than by the longer process of psychoanalysis.

The outcome of this debate will probably be that with increased knowledge we shall be able to arrive at a more accurate discrimination and diagnosis. Some mental conditions will be diagnosed as chemically based and in need of pharmacological treatment. Others will be diagnosed as both emotionally and chemically based and in need of both drug treatment and extended psychotherapy. Others again will be found to be emotionally based in the Freudian and Jungian sense and to need analytical treatment. Psychotic illnesses will probably be found to have a chemical component: neurotic conditions will probably be found to be mainly emotional and relational. There is no more place for sectarianism in this area of therapy than in the area of religion. What is needed is a greater openness and willingness on the part of all to give patient and prolonged attention to research in the endeavour to find out the way things are really. Especially do psychotherapists of particular schools need to be willing to re-examine their traditional presuppositions.

Our concern as Christian doctors and clergy is with health *and* salvation. In so far as ill-health is an impediment holding a person back from his true fulfilment we must be concerned for the improvement of our diagnostic powers so that all that can be done may be done to set people free from ill-health. On a purely secular evaluation of the human person there is still much to be done to improve our powers of diagnosis at the biological and biochemical levels no less than at the psychological and sociological. Because the priest as counsellor no less than the doctor as consultant needs to have an understanding of the totality of the human person, it is essential in the training of clergy and ministers that they should be helped to know enough about the physiological and psychological structures of personality and about the methods of medical and psy-

chotherapeutic diagnosis to be able to co-operate meaningfully.
The priest needs to know enough to be able to discriminate between
sickness of soul and sickness of mind and sickness of body. He needs
to know when to call in the help of other diagnosticians. It will not
help to offer a man spiritual advice for dealing with his irritability
if what is causing the irritability is an as yet undetected brain tumour.
That is a somewhat dramatic way of saying that the church sometimes offers spiritual advice to people who need medical or psychiatric help first. If a person is suffering from psychological illness, to
superimpose upon this a certain type of religious practice may make
that person more ill than he was before. Some kinds of religious
practice are themselves signs of emotional ill-health. If one is led to
ask why it is that a seemingly religious person is not more liberated,
more loving, it may be because underneath the 'religion' is an
undetected and undealt-with area of emotional problem of one kind
or another. Anthony Storr, in his recent book on *Human Aggression*,
explains that while aggressive energies are a necessary part of human
life, these energies can if inverted in childhood lead to all sorts of
strange paranoic attitudes and behaviour.

If then there is, as I believe, a Christian ministry to men and
women which can liberate them from partial and narrow living
into fuller, freer attitudes and relationships – and if the Christian
gospel is precisely the offer of this salvation, this liberation into
ever more mature and joyful personal living – then the minister of
this word and of these sacraments needs to be sufficiently aware of
what is known about human emotional growth and development –
about physical and psychopathic, as well as moral and spiritual
hindrances to that growth – if he is to operate effectively in his own
field as consultant and guide.

If diagnosis in the field of health is a means towards the treatment
of illness and the recovery of the capacity to fulfil one's own role
in life, diagnosis in the dimension in which the words *God* and
Faith have meaning is a means towards the treatment of those
obstacles which prevent a person from finding fulfilment and wholeness in a life oriented towards God and towards other people in and
through Christ. But because a person is a single organism of inter-
related aspects, the spiritual guide needs to have an adequate
understanding of diagnosis and treatment in the field of health.
Above all the clergy need to take seriously what the psychologists
have to tell us about the nature of the human psyche. The demands

of a real pastoral love require that we shall take all the trouble that is necessary to see that our knowledge is as good as it can be if we are to be servants of an individual's true spiritual growth. On the one hand no drug will help a person who is refusing to face up to some personal, moral problem. On the other hand a wrong diagnosis in the other sphere may increase mental illness. But this having been said, what we are ultimately concerned about as Christians is not only that sick persons shall be able to cope with the demands of life within a tolerable margin of anxiety: we are concerned to open up for men and women that 'life more abundant' of which Christ speaks – a life marked by an inward strength to cope with suffering: a life marked by a greater concern for the well-being of others, a life that has in it that buoyancy for which the Christian word is joy. The Christian vision is of a person who grows into a whole person in and through the pressures and hard necessities of life. This vision makes the highest demands of the spiritual guide as diagnostician: how is *this* person with his or her particular personality to be helped to grow from where he or she is towards that person he or she is capable of becoming by learning to be open to God and open to other persons in the given situation? This is an art of arts – of spiritual diagnosis and guidance. There is no rule book for those of us who under God are used in this way either as preachers or teachers or as spiritual consultants and guides. Each person's need is his own.

The Christian concern then is for health *and* salvation. All healing we believe is of God and we need to understand that knowledge about human nature that belongs to modern medicine. But salvation stands for a growth and enhancement of human living – a personal reorientation and redirection – a response that is more than a healthy functioning of mind and body, and may sometimes be combined with illness which has not yielded to treatment. *Health* and *salvation* are words that stand for two aspects of human growth and fulfillment: while they must not be confused, they are sufficiently related for it to be important for the minister of the gospel of salvation to be conversant with that knowledge of human nature which belongs to the biochemist, the psychotherapist and the psychologist: but his concern is for the growth and development of new men in Christ.

2 Psychiatry and Religion

James Mathers

Dr James Mathers is a Consultant Psychiatrist and Medical Superintendent of Rubery Hill Hospital, Birmingham.

This chapter is based on a lecture which he gave at a study course for younger Anglican clergy in the Diocese of Chelmsford at Severalls (Psychiatric) Hospital in September 1968.

A psychiatrist's business often lies in exploring those parts of his patient's experience which arouse feelings of fear, shame and disgust. He has to become intimately acquainted with ugliness, injustice and cruelty. At the end of one of my outpatient sessions, I happened to hear a service on the radio. The lesson was from Philippians: 'And now, my friends, all that is noble, all that is just and pure, all that is lovable and gracious, whatever is excellent and admirable – fill all your thoughts with these things' (Phil. 4.8). I found myself reflecting that while my ultimate objective, like St Paul's, was to enable men to become whole, my method of helping them seemed almost diametrically opposed to his. He recommends the contemplation of the beautiful and good, while my practice seemed to involve an almost obsessive preoccupation with the ugly and evil.

This apparent paradox has stuck in my mind, and over the years I have tried to understand the relation between these two approaches to the problem of helping men to deal with the evil parts of their experience – by focusing attention on the evil, as doctors tend to do, or by focusing attention away from evil and on to the good, as St Paul recommends.

On the whole, doctors want people to get better. They want to help them achieve, maintain or increase their health. Perhaps because it was never made explicit, the hardest lesson I learned in medical school was that health is not to be sought there, and that if perchance it was found, it was not a matter for my attention. None but the sick were to be studied – the healthy were thrown out; and I was never allowed to diagnose someone as being healthy, but was limited to the traditional cautious statement that he showed 'no apparent disease'. Over the years, I did absorb this lesson. The study of disease, and the various special or specific ways in which scientific method enabled us to attack it, was fascinating and the results often very gratifying. So I was content to follow my teachers' example, of advancing towards the objective of getting people healthy by, so to speak, walking backwards, and focusing attention only on their diseases.

After a few years of practice, of course, I realized that my training had been somewhat one-sided, and began to redress the balance from my own experience. I became aware of several conceptual or semantic confusions which obscured the problem. Let me mention two of them.

1. When we talk of treatment (or cure) we do not often make it clear whether we mean the treatment of patients or the treatment of diseases. Yet there is a great deal of difference: to treat a disease means to attack, destroy or inhibit it in some way. To treat a patient, on the other hand, means to foster, nurture or care for his capacity for living. These are quite different kinds of activity. A doctor does not try to foster, nurture or care for a disease process; nor does he try to attack, destroy or inhibit the life of his patient. Probably most of the stories of healing in the scriptures are to be interpreted as concerned with the healing of persons; while most of the advice given in modern medical textbooks is concerned with the treatment of diseases, by procedures such as sticking knives or needles or poisonous substances into people which are potentially damaging to them – though one hopes they will be more certainly damaging to their diseases.

2. Doctors use the word 'patient' for those we try to help. The word means someone who is passive. It is appropriate for someone who is anaesthetized, and sometimes for those who are consciously submitting to diagnostic procedures. It is much less often appropriate for people to whom we offer advice or prescriptions. Many so-called patients – perhaps most – decide for themselves whether they will act on the advice, or take their tablets as ordered. They are not really patients – they are *agents*; and to expect them to continue to behave passively and obediently is unrealistic and confusing.

Perhaps there is a similar confusion in our understanding of the scriptures, which I can illustrate by contrasting the saying of Jesus, 'unless you become like children, you will never enter the Kingdom of Heaven' (Matt. 18.3) – with St Paul's repeated emphasis upon the necessity for the Christian to become a mature man, to 'put away childish things' (1 Cor. 13.11; 14.20; Col. 1.28; Heb. 5.12). We have to choose, from moment to moment, whether the child, trustingly dependent on a parent-figure, or the man in his maturity (perfection), expresses more appropriately the ideal of spiritual health. Just as theologians are currently contemplating the idea of 'man come of age' as against the idea of man as a 'child of God', so perhaps doctors have to face the fact that their patients, if they are to regain their health, must also become agents in their own recovery. Both spiritual and mental health require that a man should be able to accept and exercise responsibility.

It is, of course, in the understanding of disease that scientific method has been so successful. In many instances it enables doctors to know what specific mechanism or structure is defective, and to know what therapeutic measure is therefore indicated. But scientific method does not help to get the sufferer to accept the prescription offered. It helps understanding but not treatment. Unless the sufferer is unconscious, or unless we use brute force, this remains a function of the personal relationship, a matter of asserting authority, or persuasion, or cajolery or trickery. You can take a horse to the water but you cannot make him drink.

In psychiatry, scientific method has not yet led to any major breakthrough in our understanding of specific disease processes except in a very few instances, and most of our organic treatments are non-specific. We shock people out of their symptoms or we blunt their capacity for expressing or feeling emotion. Instead of using snakepits or mandragora we use ECT or synthetic tranquillizers but otherwise we have not got far. But if our repertory of treatment for disease remains fairly primitive, we have begun to make a little progress in our ideas about the treatment of people. Somewhere towards the end of the eighteenth century there began to be practised so-called 'moral treatment', a humanely inspired movement based on the principle that even if a man had lost his reason, he could only learn to behave responsibly again if he were treated as a responsible person. The therapy emphasized 'close and friendly association with the patient, intimate discussion of his difficulties, and the daily pursuit of purposeful activity'.[1] 'It was a way of life offered to the sick, under the direction of physicians whose philosophy of mental illness was based on a high valuation of the individual and belief in his recuperative powers.'[2]

Moral treatment was, of course, a treatment of the person, enhancing his capacity for health, so that the disease from which he suffered became less overwhelming. It had a general effect, which could benefit anyone whatever specific disease he might have.

It gradually fell into disuse through the second half of the last century and the first half of the twentieth partly because of the rising enthusiasm which doctors felt for the scientific attack on disease which was proving so successful in other fields. This meant that patients were regarded merely as vehicles for the diseases, which were the real focus of interest. It might not have mattered too much had the scientific attack on disease in the psychiatric field been rapidly successful; but it was not. And the outcome of the neglect of the person which resulted from focusing only on his disease was entirely disastrous, allowing the monstrous growth of depersonalizing and harmful institutions which are such an impediment to our efforts to help people today.

In this second half of the twentieth century we are trying to redress the balance. One of Freud's greatest contributions to our understanding of persons was his focusing of attention on the relationship which grows up between the sufferer and the therapist – what he spoke of as transference and counter-transference. From this original emphasis for therapy on the relationship between two people has slowly emerged the whole flowering of what we now call human relations – from individual psychotherapy, on the one hand to the manifold kinds of casework and counselling professions, and on the other hand to group therapy, so-called therapeutic communities, and what has been called administrative therapy. The understanding of human relations has also affected many of the ways in which we practise so-called rehabilitation, after-care or resocialization – though perhaps not yet enough. All these efforts at treatment focus on the person in his relation with other persons, rather than on the disease from which he suffers.

It is much easier to relate this kind of treatment of persons, this kind of health-enhancing activity, to the kind of teaching about love of the brethren which we find in the Christian gospel than it is to relate the scientific attack on disease to it. Paul Halmos has shown, in his book *The Faith of the Counsellors*[3], how difficult it is to separate the objectives and values of the professional case-worker from those of the theologically oriented pastor of souls.

You can see how these two kinds of treatment seem to lead in opposite directions. If you focus attention on the disease, the person who suffers from it is a mere background to your field of study. You focus attention on a bit of him, and ignore the rest. You analyse, cut a bit out or take away a sample, and refine methods of studying the bit ever more minutely. You get to know more and more about less and less. Your doctors become more and more specialized, so that ultimately the unfortunate human being who carries the disease finds himself a lost soul, severed from all those personal relationships with his family and friends which make him human, admitted to the modern Tower of Babel, the big general hospital.

But if you focus on the person, you respect his relationships with his social surroundings. Maybe you start off by seeing him in the privacy of the consulting room, but you find that his relationships with other people have too great an influence, for good or ill, for you to ignore them. So you have to *widen* your field of study to include the sufferer's family, or his working group, or his fellow-sufferers in the ward. Inevitably, your pursuit of this method exacts its own price. Because you do not focus on his disease, you do not know so much about it, and may miss seeing details which you would see if you were just the objective scientific observer. As your field of concern gets wider, your control over the situation gets less and less, and you tend to feel powerless. But you follow this approach because it seems to lead the sufferer back to health, back to being an agent instead of a patient, to being more responsible – in spite of your inability to control the situation, and your inability to write a convincing scientific paper on how you cured him.

Another very important difference between the two approaches is that on the one hand the doctor tries to be the detached, dispassionate observer carefully excluding himself from his field of study; while on the other, since he is in relationship with the sufferer, the therapist himself is involved in the field he is studying – he is a *participant* observer, sharing in the sufferer's situation in a way which is compassionate rather than dispassionate. Certainly he has to learn to control his involvement with the sufferer's feelings, but equally certainly, he must become involved if his health-enhancing approach is to be successful.

Observe also how, while the single-minded but narrowly focussed attack on disease leads to greater and greater specialization of the doctor's role, the health-enhancing approach through fostering good relationships leads away from specialization: what began as a highly esoteric activity in the consulting rooms of the pioneer psychoanalysts is now the concern of case-workers, nurses, welfare officers and counsellors of many other kinds; while in the hospital, lay administrators are likely to find themselves in the therapeutic community meeting; and in the factory, the foreman is likely to find himself attending a course on human relations. This generalizing process is not to be seen merely as one of diluting professional skills because of the shortage of trained experts. It results from an entirely realistic acknowledgement of the significance of different people in the pattern of relationships which is of importance to the client's health. The foreman can be far more influential for a man's health than a psychiatrist or counsellor who only sees him for an hour or so once a week – or less.

Having spent so much time considering the differences between the disease-attacking approach and the health-enhancing approach to treatment, you may feel, as a good many people have suggested, that it is justifiable to establish a corresponding separation between those who practise one approach from those who practise the other. Medical practitioners might be regarded as those who specialize in the attack on disease, while psychotherapists and other non-medical counsellors specialize in the health-enhancing approach. Paul Halmos certainly excludes most doctors from his list of the counselling professions, though I am relieved to see that he includes psychiatrists.

But we should not do this too readily. Most doctors do in fact have to practise the health-enhancing relationship approach to treatment a very great deal, when they cannot find any useful specific measure to attack the disease. Although they do not learn much about it in medical school they soon learn something of it by experience. And most of the non-medical counsellors, conversely, work for agencies which try to meet a particular need for their clients, 'attacking' and trying to get rid of a particular social disability rather than offering entirely general support. So I think it is wiser for doctors and counsellors of all kinds to live with the tension involved in trying to use both approaches to their work. In any therapeutic encounter, it may at one moment be appropriate to attack the disease and at another to do something health enhancing: perhaps much of the art of helping people lies in deciding between the two from moment to moment. The relation between a person and his disease is like that between a figure and its background in a silhouette. The artist can alter the shape of the figure, or make an opposite alteration in the shape of the background, to achieve the same result.

If we think of these two approaches from a historic or evolutionary viewpoint, rather than in terms of an antithesis as we have been describing them here and now, we can begin to see that the generalized, indefinite business of health enhancement through relationship is much the more primitive and more fundamental. It is perhaps closely akin to the way we care for young children, so as to enable them to grow up to maturity. The fundamental aim of caring for people is to enable them to become whole; and the development of scientific methods of attacking disease, with its precision and clarity and predictability, is seen to be a second-order activity, developed as a valuable tool in order to achieve the same ultimate purpose. The attack on disease is a means of becoming whole, but it should not be allowed to become an end in itself. To put the point in another way: the ultimate purpose of caring for people is to enable them to achieve their optimal health; and this provides a context within which all disease-attacking procedures, as well as health-enhancing ones, have to be seen and judged.

This leads to my final point. What, after all, is health? A man is not healthy if he is badly adjusted to his environment (which includes his social environment – other people). And if his environment is itself unhealthy, as is usually the case, he is not healthy if he is well adjusted to it. He could only be perfectly healthy if he were well adjusted to a perfectly healthy environment. This is not likely to obtain except in the kingdom of heaven. So all our human notions of health must be understood as dynamic, as movement towards an optimum which is more or less remote from present reality. And this implies that we need a direction in which to move, and a goal to aim at. It is this, I think, that it is the real function of religion to provide. Medical science is only concerned with what is, not what ought to be. The norms which it uses are average measurements, not optimal ones except where the two coincide. Normal body temperature, 37°C, is both average and optimal; but normal intelligence (IQ 100) is only average. What is normal human nature? The medical scientist does not attempt to answer; but the theologian will affirm his faith that normal human nature is best exemplified by Jesus of Nazareth, the man for others, man in relationship. And since we are all to some extent men in relationship, we can only move in a healthy direction if all men are moving towards the same goal. As Christians this means, I take it, that we cannot move faster towards spiritual health than those who reject us. Love your enemies – not merely out of blind obedience to an unrealistic commandment, but because only so will we make any progress towards the kingdom.

Many of you will no doubt be concerned to fit yourselves to offer pastoral counselling to your troubled parishioners. You will be asking yourselves, when you see a person in trouble, 'What can we do to help this person?' I do not want to discourage you from this, but I must warn you of the danger of Samaritanism – of waiting until someone is half dead, thoroughly a patient, before you concern yourself with him. Most people in trouble are partly patients, and partly agents, and as such the relevant question may be 'What is this person's proper role in our joint endeavour to realize the kingdom of heaven on earth?' So many of the sick and disabled, and so many who are not so labelled, suffer or are ineffectual because they feel useless. They lack a sense of purpose. And if you have this question in mind, you may sometimes help people to see their purpose in life more clearly. I do not of course mean that you have to discuss religion with them. Often you have to be content with more immediate objectives – 'what does he want to get better for?'; or, 'what will he do with himself when he has recovered?' But for us, the guiding principle was laid down in the gospel: 'Set your mind on God's kingdom and his justice before everything else, and all the rest will come to you as well.'

NOTES

1. M. Greenblatt, R. H. York and E. L. Brown, *From Custodial to Therapeutic Patient Care in Mental Hospitals*, Russell Sage Foundation, New York, 1955, p. 407.

2. Ibid, p. 411.

3. P. Halmos, *The Faith of the Counsellors*, Constable 1965

3 The Context of Anxiety

James Mathers

Dr James Mathers is a Consultant Psychiatrist and Medical Superintendent of Rubery Hill Hospital, Birmingham.

This chapter is based on a paper read at the Annual Conference of the Institute of Religion and Medicine at Sheffield in July 1967.

The problem of trying to understand what another person means is really that of being able to share the other's experience. Such sharing of experience can never be more than partial, on the one hand because we are separate individuals, and on the other because we can only get to know about the other's experience by perceiving his behaviour; and all too frequently this is misinterpreted. The professional skill of the psychiatrist is concerned more with understanding the ways in which our behaviour distorts the meaning of our experience than with any special intuitive ability to understand another's experience itself.

In this paper I want to talk not as a psychiatrist, concerned with the mechanisms of distortion of self-expression, but as an ordinary human being trying to understand the experience of anxiety which everyone has at times. To do this I am going to compare the meaning which the experience of anxiety might have for three different individuals – a new-born baby, a child of three or four years old, and the historical figure of Jesus. Clearly this is an exercise of imagination and guesswork, but it may help to suggest how the experience of anxiety can have a different meaning for persons at different stages of development; and I hope it may provide some kind of a bridge between the scientific viewpoint, concerned with anxiety as it is, and the religious or theological viewpoint, which I take to be concerned with anxiety as it ought to be (or ought not to be).

First, let us consider another kind of experience in which both doctors and theologians have a particular interest. This is the particular form of the anxiety experience which we recognize as a sense of guilt. Whereas anxiety (the experience of a 'numbing loneliness, isolation and disorganization of experience', as Erikson[1] describes it), is aroused in earliest infancy, when instinctual desires are frustrated by mother's apparent absence, a sense of guilt can only be differentiated from it after the small child has developed the beginnings of conscience – when its innate desires are frustrated by the internalized prohibitions of parent-figures (super-ego).

Both anxiety and the sense of guilt carry the same basic meaning, of a threat to the individual's ego-identity or self-esteem.[2] It is the task of psychopathology to elucidate the various mechanisms by which the human being, consciously or unconsciously, tries to evade these very unpleasant experiences – mechanisms such as denial, projection, displacement, dissociation and so on. Such mental mechanisms are still apparently accepted as pathological: in fact, they very often seem to be pretty effective and they appear to be universal among the species, so it is rather surprising that someone has not suggested their recategorization as psychophysiological rather than psychopathological. I suppose this is because of an unspoken awareness that, although they may be 'normal' in the sense of being average, they are not normal in the proper sense of being optimal. Perhaps the clergy recognize more readily than the psychopathologist that there is another, more difficult way for a man to deal with his sense of guilt – an optimal way, which is not unconscious and is not automatic. This is by experiencing repentance – *metanoia* – a change of mind. It is characteristic of this change of mind that it is in the direction of reconciliation (with God and one's brethren); which is to say that it leads away from an egocentric context to a sociocentric or God-centred one. The man no longer judges his guilty act or guilty state as something for which he, alone and unaided, has to accept responsibility, but recognizes that, being restored to communion with his fellows, the responsibility for his state and his behaviour is now something he shares with them. And similarly, of course, he finds that he is expected to accept some responsibility for the state and behaviour of his fellows.

I want to examine the possibility that the optimal way for a man to deal with the anxiety experience is also through a change of mind, a *metanoia*, of a similar kind. The word 'repentance' can be defined as a 'change from past evil'; so when the psychotherapist seeks to help his client to 'work through' his anxiety, is he really helping him to 'repent' from his anxiety?

Let me make some preliminary comments. Firstly, I am talking primarily about subjective experience, anxiety, and only incidentally about objectively observable phenomena. But I shall assume that anxiety always affects behaviour, however deviously; and that this behaviour can be observed and interpreted by others. (I acknowledge that the behaviour of one person is frequently unobserved or misunderstood by others but, in principle, I consider that a man cannot help expressing his experience by his behaviour except for short periods, and when he panics. Panic, of course, is the most severe form of anxiety, and its main behavioural characteristic is that its expression conveys confusing signals or no signals for communication to others. However, this does not prevent its *being* communicated, since the mere absence of signals from another person who is seen to be alive is anxiety-provoking.)

Secondly, we must be clear that we are concerned with neurotic anxiety, and that this is an experience directly rooted in the infant's experience of dread, antedating that stage of development when the infant can locate the source of the threat.[3] It is therefore more primitive than fear of an objectively perceived danger (whether located inside or outside the body). It is free-floating anxiety – the fear of non-being. Anxiety is rearoused in later life by any situation which is subjectively perceived as a crisis – that is, by a situation presenting a problem which previous experience, guidance or education has not equipped the individual to solve; and this later experience of anxiety inevitably draws its patterning and quality, and to a variable extent its vehemence – from all previous experiences of anxiety back to infancy. However much the current crisis may differ in externals from former ones, the neurotic anxiety experience is the same one – it has, so to speak, an identity, even if it alters; just as I am still the same person as I was when I was a child, even though I differ in certain respects from what I was then, and might not be recognized from my photograph.

Thirdly, we are concerned with what is potential in the human phenomenon rather than what is actual. For this reason, and because we are focusing on a subjective experience, the traditional methods of objective science cannot be expected to test the validity of my hypothesis. In Teilhard de Chardin's words, we are concerned with the 'within' rather than the 'without' of things.[4]

When a baby experiences anxiety it expresses distress, and mother is moved to behave in such a way as to reassure it. What moves her to do so? It is clearly something much more primitive than a rational decision. Her motive is not properly described as altruistic. It is compassionate – a fellow-feeling. She shares in the child's anxiety in some degree. If she feels nothing of this, she does nothing; and indeed, if she behaves with irritation or rejection, it is only because she cannot help feeling anxiety in response to the baby's cry – though her behaviour is inappropriate. The behaviour she usually exhibits is thus directed to the relief of the anxiety of both the baby and herself. Her reassurance relieves the baby of the feeling that his existence is threatened, and in so doing she enables his sense of personal identity to grow stronger. The basic strength of the human infant, according to Erikson, is hope; 'the enduring belief in the attainability of fervent wishes, in spite of the dark urges and rages which mark the beginning of existence.'[5]

There are of course many situations in which mother no sooner perceives the child's anxiety than she is able, through her superior ability, to abolish it forthwith by unilateral action. Such unilateral behaviour by a parent-figure confirms and validates the infant's hopefulness; and at this early stage it may be all the child needs to continue healthy development. Similarly, in the doctor/patient encounter, the doctor's diagnostic skill and therapeutic experience may justify his prescription of treatment with only a trivial degree of emotional involvement or compassion.

But hope is only the first of the virtues or strengths which a person needs to develop if he is to master later anxieties. Erikson lists eight of them, each emerging as the attainment of successive stages of development. After *hope* in infancy come *will*, *purpose* and *competence* in childhood; *fidelity* marks the emergence from adolescence, and mutual *love*, *care* for dependents, and ultimately *wisdom*, are the virtues of adult life.

So let us move on a little, to a stage when the child has clearly gained an awareness of self, and is mastering his wilfulness. (Will is 'the unbroken determination to exercise free choice as well as self-restraint, in spite of the unavoidable experience of shame and doubt in infancy'.[6]) At such a stage it is probable that mother will sometimes reassure her child by saying 'we don't feel so frightened (or angry or anxious) do we?' She uses the first person plural. It seems that the child is now able to experience himself as part of a group of two – a group which, so to speak, experiences anxiety mainly 'in' him. So the context of the anxiety experience is altered: from being a threat to the child's ego-identity pure and simple, it becomes partly at least a threat to a 'we'-identity. And the responsibility for the solution of the child's problem is experienced as being not 'mine alone' but 'mine as a member of this group'.

At this stage, it is clear that the childish virtues of will, purpose or competence (whichever is appropriate) will not be adequately exercized and confirmed if the parent always relieves the anxiety aroused by every new crisis by unilateral action (if she 'wraps the child in cotton wool'). Having enabled her child to experience his anxiety in a 'we'-context, she has to begin posing the question 'how will we solve this problem?', so that the child can begin to take on the responsibility of group membership by adding his own initiative to the solution. In this way, crisis becomes the occasion of learning, and progress towards maturity can proceed.

Having had a brief look at what may potentially happen to the child's experience of anxiety, we must consider what is involved for the mother or parent-figure who tries to help. We can note first of all that if someone is to be relieved of anxiety in an optimal way, there does have to be another person who cares. (In everyday life, no doubt many sufferers are left to cope with anxiety more or less on their own; and usually this results in the development of psychopathological symptoms by the action of unconscious defence mechanisms – as, for instance, Freud demonstrated in his *Psychopathology of Everyday Life*. Possibly, older children whose ego-strength is in any case likely to be increasing through the general processes of physical and emotional growth, might occasionally learn to solve new and critical problems on their own, without the current support of a caring person; but for them to do so without developing some quirk of character or behaviour which betrays the presence of an unresolved anxiety must be rare.)

To respond to an anxious person's signals of distress by caring for him is not an inescapable biological imperative. Certainly, it is common enough in maternal experience; but as we saw, mother's behaviour is directed as much to relieving her own anxiety, aroused by the child's distress, as it is to relieving the child's distress itself. Anxiety is catching, and its expression is repellent rather than attractive. Unless there is a prior bond of love or commitment to an anxious person, most of us will try to avoid him, or seek a quick escape from the infection of anxiety. If we do not literally cross the road to avoid him, we find ourselves remembering an urgent appointment, or we buy the sufferer a drink, and perhaps have one ourselves. In the consulting room, the doctor or psychiatrist finds himself prescribing a sedative instead of making time to listen to the patient's story.

But in my own case, for instance, I do have a professional commitment to the anxious person; and however much my immediate reaction may be to escape from the contagion of anxiety, the very fact that the sufferer has appealed to me for help means that my self-esteem is jeopardized if I fail to help him; and since it is often the case that, as an onlooker, I can see possibilities of solving his problem which have not occurred to him, there is a conflict between my desire to escape and my desire to help. This experience appears basically similar to that of the mother with her child. But, as we have seen, once the child has achieved a separate ego-identity, the unilateral solving of the critical problem by mother denies the child a necessary learning experience; and the same difficulty arises in any care-giving or therapeutic situation.

For the helping person, therefore, the implications of all this seem to be that he must be able to form a bond with the sufferer so that together they form a 'we'-group; and that he must (temporarily) have the ability to experience and tolerate the other's anxiety until he understands, and until the sufferer also understands, how the problem may be solved; and he must have the strength not to allow himself to use psychopathological mechanisms to cut short the process.

So far so good. But what are we to say about the situation when the helper sees no solution to the problem presented by the anxious one; or, if he thinks he sees it, finds that the solution lies far outside the competence of either of them? This is the common experience of social workers and social psychiatrists. The 'we'-group of two, helper and sufferer, is a context which is too narrow for most real-life situations other than that of mother and infant. We find that all the members of a family, or primary group, tend to be involved in the anxiety and crisis of the individual; and in turn, we find that the crises and problems of families and primary groups are themselves involved in those of the community at large. Some of us, committed either professionally or through love of our fellows, have learned to tolerate some of the anxieties of individuals; and some fewer of us are beginning to learn the harder task of tolerating the anxieties of families and small groups. Some of R. D. Laing's recent essays[7] show what a hard task this can be. But how many of us can look at the anxiety and panic of our whole generation without escaping into psychopathology?

You will remember that we are looking for optimal ways of dealing with anxiety rather than average, pathological ways. The value of an optimum is that it can sometimes be a true norm – a fixed standard by which we can evaluate, if not measure, the sub-optimal phenomena of experience and behaviour with which we are in daily contact. Stephen Neill has made the point that in this proper sense of the word, normal human nature is best exemplified by Jesus of Nazareth.[8]

Let us consider what may have been his experience of anxiety. Since he was fully human, he no doubt had infantile and childhood experiences of it but we cannot usefully guess at them. We can guess that in his baptism he was affirming his common humanity and his willingness to share in the anxieties of his fellows (which, as we have seen, is a primary condition of ability to help others). His experience in the wilderness must at the least have exercised his capacity for withstanding anxiety; and indeed, we can see, in the account of the temptations, how the devil invited him to evade the challenge of affirming his true self, his sense of identity, by sub-optimal techniques – or mental mechanisms.

During his ministry we are told of several occasions on which he went apart from the multitudes. No doubt, as the records say, he went apart to pray, but we can guess that these would be times when he felt that 'virtue had gone out of him'. This is a common enough human experience and we can fill it out a bit. When we have this feeling, at the end of a session when we have been involving our-selves in caring for anxious people, what does it mean to us? That we feel exhausted, emotionally drained. We become irritable and uncertain of our judgment. If circumstances forced us to carry on without rest or refreshment to our spirit, we would feel that our ego-identity, our self-esteem would be threatened. In fact we would suffer, albeit transiently, from anxiety.

Jesus cared for individuals, sharing their anxieties as a parent. Surely he suffered from this shared anxiety. His ministry to indi-viduals led him to criticize the scribes and Pharisees – the social establishment of his day, which, as always in human history rejects and excommunicates those whose anxieties it finds intolerable. And then, when his experience of the social factors underlying individuals' anxieties was ripe, he went up to Jerusalem, to the seat of the temporal and ecclesiastical power. He wept over it; and thereafter followed the experience in Gethsemane and the crucifixion.

What are we to think of his experience in Gethsemane? Throughout his ministry he had shared the anxieties of those who had sought his aid. He had risen above the temptations to escape from anxiety by magical (dissociative) means (making stones into bread), or by using worldly power, or by a self-destroying gesture (by throwing himself down from the temple parapet). In going to Jerusalem he faced the ultimate challenge to his self-evaluation as the bringer of Life, God's Messiah. In the garden he experienced 'horror and dismay', and his 'heart was ready to break with grief'. Was this because he was afraid of the cross, afraid of personal death? Or was it because the load of anxiety and sense of guilt which he had so willingly shared with the rest of humanity had become too great to be borne by one human being?

Such an attempt as this to guess at the vicissitudes of another person's subjective experience makes clear the inadequacy of our language for the purpose. I started with a definition of anxiety as meaning a threat to *ego*-identity or *self*-esteem. When discussing anxiety in the growing child I talked of its becoming, at least partly, a threat to a 'we'-identity; and now I find myself talking of the experience of Jesus as that of anxiety, though here we must guess that its meaning was his fear lest chaos should continue to be the lot of that humanity with which he had identified himself, his fear that his prayer 'that they may all be one' should remain unanswered, or answered negatively.

I am not happy to be using the same word for these three very different experiences. But they seem to have an identity in the same way that the words infant, boy, adolescent, man can all be used of the same individual. The three different experiences are really, perhaps, the same experience in the context of different stages of development.

Let me finally go back to the question I posed at the beginning. Is the problem of 'working through' anxiety really the same as the problem of 'repenting' from a sense of guilt? I would suggest that it is. Since a sense of guilt is a derivative of anxiety, this would not be improbable on *a priori* grounds. It seems to me that the change of context, from ego-identity through successive stages of 'we'-identity, are each of them occasions for *metanoia*, for a change of mind, in each of which anxiety is experienced in a new perspective, each leading forward to a greater maturity, a great integrity of personality, and – paradox of life itself – to a readiness to accept ever greater burdens and thus risk the new-found integrity anew.

NOTES

1. E. H. Erikson, *Childhood and Society*, Hogarth Press, 2nd ed. 1963, p. 20
2. E. H. Erikson, *Insight and Responsibility*, Faber and Faber 1964, p. 86
3. S. Freud, *Introductory Lectures on Psychoanalysis*, Allen & Unwin, 2nd ed. 1943, p. 341
4. P. Teilhard de Chardin, *The Phenomenon of Man*, Collins 1959, p. 53 ff.
5. E. H. Erikson, *Insight and Responsibility*, p. 118
6. Ibid., p. 119
7. R. D. Laing, *The Politics of Experience*, Penguin Books 1967
8. S. Neill, *A Genuinely Human Existence*, Constable & Co. 1959, p. 35

4 Conflicts and Anxieties of the Patient Seeking Healing

I. B. Sneddon

Dr Sneddon is Consultant Dermatologist and Director of Clinical Studies in the University of Sheffield.

This chapter is based on a talk given at a Conference in July 1967 at Sheffield for doctors, clergy, and social workers entitled 'Conflicts and Anxieties of Patients and their Helpers'.

Anxiety in patients seeking healing is no new problem. Pliny the Elder in the early years AD wrote, 'It is unfortunate that there is no law to punish ignorant physicians. They learn by our suffering and they experiment by putting us to death.' Even the effect of clinical teaching of students on the patient, a highly topical subject, was summed up in an epigram by Martial the Roman poet (I give the English translation for the benefit of those who would miss the point if I quoted the original):

> I am ill. I send for Symmachus: he's here,
> A hundred students following in the rear.
> All paw my chest with hands as cold as snow.
> I had no fever but I have it now.

Thus the problem of patients appear to have been much the same over the years, but recently there has been more discontent amongst patients complaining of the inadequacies of their doctor, and doctors complaining about the demands of their patients.

I am going to try, if possible, to discuss some of the problems which patients have, as seen by the hospital doctor. It is a subject which has interested me since so often I realize that even after great efforts have been made to help them, some patients leave hospital disappointed by what has been achieved. Firstly, what brings the patient to the doctor? With exception of accidents and acute emergencies that arise so quickly there is hardly time to become

B

anxious, the majority of patients are driven to their doctor by fear. Sometimes these are rational, sometimes irrational, the latter being the more difficult to dispel. Fear of death, fear of pain, fear of cancer, fear of contagion or venereal disease, fear of mental disease, fear of pregnancy, fear of anaesthetics, fear of hospitals: the fears are endless.

Many of them can be dealt with only if they are recognized by the doctor, since they may not be voiced by the patient. Some months ago I saw a man who came to me because a friend of his had recently developed cancer of the lip, and my patient, feeling round his own mouth with his tongue, found a rough area inside one cheek, and naturally assumed that he had a cancer too. The rough patch had, in fact, been present for many years, but had never been drawn to his attention before he heard about his friend's illness. Fortunately the condition was a harmless one, but nevertheless this was a rational fear.

Some weeks after this, a miserable, rather spotty youth came in to my out-patients complaining of headache, aching in his joints, tiredness and a rash on his face and shoulders. Examination revealed only that he had a mild adolescent acne, and this would not account for his many symptoms. I asked him what he thought was the matter, and he said he was sure he had got syphilis. When asked why, he said he had been idly turning the leaves of a medical book at home, and had come across the section of syphilis and started to read it. Syphilis, he read, presented with a rash frequently pustular, headache and pains all over the body. This boy only had acne and an irrational fear.

Many of the fears which bring our patients are far more difficult to unearth, and the doctor has to divine them because the patient may well not bring them out openly. This is particularly so of fear and symptoms based on sexual abnormalities, and these may not be discussed with the family doctor, because the patient knows him too well. He does not like discussing what may be a moral problem with someone whose respect he wishes to keep. I often see patients who prefer to unburden themselves to a relative stranger at a hospital clinic rather than to tell their well-loved family doctor.

There are, therefore, patients who complain of symptoms which are apparently trivial, yet which may be an excuse to get to the doctor's surgery so that their underlying fears may be set at rest. If the consultation is conducted too expeditiously the patient will never get round to voicing his fears. Balint, I think, has stressed the fact that the patient should be encouraged to talk and not to answer questions. It is always my practice to ask a patient what he thinks is the matter. One gets some extraordinarily funny answers but quite often one gets the truth. One of the problems of achieving successful treatment is persuading the patient to consent to having the appropriate treatment. Although one may recognize that the patient requires psychiatric treatment, a certain number of patients will refuse to see a psychiatrist. Certainly in the North of England, to the more primitive of our patients, the psychiatrist is the man with the evil eye, and even when in a hospital clinic we have disguised a psychiatrist as a dermatologist, the subterfuge has quickly been detected, and the patient has refused to co-operate. I feel that this fear of psychotherapy is one reason why those who are depressed may not reach help in time.

Another problem is to persuade a patient that hospital admission, which may be essential, is accepted. Tempers may well get frayed when the doctor tries to persuade a patient who requires treatment, to be admitted, and the patient appears to be stupid when he will not accept obviously good advice. Sometimes it is due to sheer animal fear of the unknown, sometimes fear of anaesthesia rather than the surgical procedure, sometimes fear of surgery. As far as admission to a medical side of a hospital is concerned, a mere explanation as to what is going to take place may get over the difficulty of the fear of anaesthetics or surgery. It may well be related to things outside hospital. Women will not come in sometimes because they do not trust their husbands to remain faithful while they are in hospital. Women also feel a loss of face if they cannot cope with their housework and have to hand over their home to someone else. Recently I had great difficulty in persuading a woman who was obviously ill and incapable of continuing at home, to come in, because she felt that her husband and son could not manage without her. While they might not keep up the same standard of hygiene that she had, they managed well, and within forty-eight hours of admission to hospital the woman was feeling better, and she appreciated that the right decision had been taken.

There are those who also hate the lack of privacy in hospitals, including the old lady who recently refused to come in because she wore a wig and was afraid that this would be discovered by the anaesthetist when she had her anaesthetic.

Although one obviously cannot question the principle of publicizing things that go wrong in hospital, too much play by the press on the very small percentage of mistakes adds to the fears of the patient. Only the other day I tried to persuade an old gentleman to come in to hospital, but his reason for refusal was that we were sure to take the wrong leg off if we were going to cut one off, this fear having been produced by reading the daily press a few days before.

Once the patient has been admitted to hospital, he is in a strange and alien community. Even those of us who work in hospital get easily lost and confused when we go to visit another hospital, and one's attitude to the institution may well depend on one's first contact with the people who work there. Unhelpful, rude, brusque handling by porters, or even consultants, in the front corridor, may alter the whole attitude of the patient who is being admitted. Once, perhaps not very safely tucked in a hospital bed, life, I imagine, must be very strange. The labelling of personnel in hospital with badges which say who they are, has, I should think, helped, but there are still very many people who come to the bedside with little preliminary explanation as to why they have come, who may confuse the patient. As well as the nurses and medical staff who presumably are fairly easily recognizable, there may well be medical social workers, laboratory technicians, ECG technicians, radiographers, dieticians, medical students, physiotherapists. It is really quite endless. And I am afraid, in the flurry and obvious pressure which there is on a busy hospital, the patient may not have everything fully explained to him.

Not very long ago I admitted a woman for the investigation of what I knew was a relatively harmless skin condition. I had thought that this message had got over to her. However, during the process of some investigations which were fairly elaborate and searching, we watched the patient become more and more silent and withdrawn, and eventually Sister said to me, 'Do you know what's the matter with Mrs So-and-so'. I said, 'No'. She said, 'Well, the patient thinks that you are looking for a cancer.' This had, in fact, never been a possibility and I had not visualized that the patient would have thought that we were looking for this. She had therefore spent four or five utterly wretched days which could easily have been dealt with much earlier had we had the insight into what was worrying her.

Now this leads me on to the question of how much to tell, and who is to do it. But if you tell, how much does the patient understand or remember? I think it fair to say that few people would deliberately withhold information to a patient if they thought that uncertainty was going to lead to anxiety, but many of us have little time to explain things at great length, and this undoubtedly leads to one of the biggest troubles of patients, which is voiced over and over again. 'They never tell me anything!' There are so many reasons why this arises. Firstly, under the existing system where we have a firm of doctors headed by a consultant, senior registrar, registrar, houseman, carrying out ward rounds in public with students, only the most forthright and uninhibited patient will want to discuss intimate problems in this environment. Those patients who perhaps most need to talk will remain silent. Thus their fears and frustrations mount up. I think that, although accepting that there is a difficulty in communication, often patients are told and do not listen or do not understand. To give you a light-hearted example. For many years we have been treating women patients who develop an allergy to the nickel of their suspenders, and they recover if they will cast away these suspenders and wear substitute ones of another material. One realizes how few take this message in by the number who, after having explained allergy and all about it to them, turn round and say, 'Are you sure it isn't a germ, doctor?' Others go on their way, and you think you have got the message across, to find they come back months later, not improved, still wearing their nickel suspenders. In fact we have reached such a stage of desperation about this element of communication that we now stock in our department nylon suspender buckles. We thrust them in the patients' hands and say, 'Stitch these on your corsets and you will never have a rash again.' I do not therefore always believe when a patient says, 'They never told me.'

A very wise general practitioner friend of mine always writes down the salient features of his advice and gives it to the patient on a piece of paper to read afterwards. By far the best way of communicating with the patient is for the doctor who is really in charge of the case to explain step by step what is happening. But by the very nature of things this is impossible in a great many cases and some other substitute for the doctor in charge has to do it. Often the ward sister who takes his place may be excellent and serves both as ward sister, adviser and doctor. Sometimes a house physician or house surgeon is particularly effective, but one has to remember they are young, inexperienced, and they cannot be expected to be always wise. The medical social worker and the chaplain can do a great deal, but there is really no adequate substitute for the personal doctor with whom the patient can have a private discussion. Even so I am constantly amazed at the implicit trust the patients have in their doctors. Frequently they will allow themselves to be opened and filleted of many of their organs without really asking what is going to be done, or what has been done, and despite all the criticism which is at present aimed at the health services, the general public still have great confidence that what is done for them has been carefully considered and planned, and all is done for the best. In most cases it has, and the only weak link in the chain of communication is the last step to the patient.

One must constantly remember that patients are exposed also to information from other sources than the correct ones. Not long ago a friend of mine was an in-patient awaiting a relatively trivial eye investigation and, when seen one day reading the newspaper by the ward cleaner, the cleaner said to her, 'That's right, luv, read whilst you can.' And some patients may be cruel to each other. Not very long ago a young patient of mine suffering from a malignant growth was informed of this fact by another patient. Quite how the other patient got the news I do not know, but there is always a grapevine in the ward.

I have said nothing as yet about the effect of hospital admission itself on the patient. I never cease to be surprised at the way most people accept conditions which are quite alien to their own surroundings. Ordered about to some extent; fed on possibly unpalatable and probably unfamiliar food; kept awake by other noisy sleepers, banging trolleys and noisy lifts; sometimes faced with unpleasant sights and sounds with which normally they would never come in contact; the majority of patients adjust remarkably well and become integrated into a new group in a ward full of patients. This integration into a group is itself a great difficulty. One's status in the ward, unlike that in life outside, depends not on external trappings such as one's car or a job, or house or smart clothes, but on one's ability to fit in. One therefore has to make a position anew in the community, and this may not be easy, particularly for the elderly.

Many of us, when we are ill, desire silence and to be left alone, and this is almost impossible in a general ward. Our hospitals are woefully equipped with so-called amenity beds which give some privacy, and I would have thought that the patient's lot could be made much happier if we had more opportunities of allowing patients to be in small bedded units. This is, of course, envisaged for most new hospitals, but there has been so little building as yet.

Perhaps I should finish on the question of the patient who becomes too well integrated into the hospital ward. We have all become familiar with those who use the hospital as a shelter against life's troubles. Many patients subconsciously, if not consciously, are aware that hospital is literally a refuge and do not wish to face the outside world again. This accounts for the many patients who, when they have heard that they are about to be discharged, have a severe recurrence of symptoms, an everyday occurrence in every ward.

One must always remember that it does require courage to face the outside world again. Life is strange outside, and this is yet another of the conflicts which may face the patient who has successfully adjusted to the admission to hospital. Despite all the criticisms, they have been surrounded by people who care for them, and they are loathe to face the world without the support of their helpers.

5 Anxiety and Authority in a Therapeutic Community

J. S. Cox

The Reverend John Cox became interested in the question of authority in a therapeutic community as the result of a two-term appointment at the John Conolly Hospital, Birmingham. He was then a student on the Diploma in Pastoral Studies course under Dr Lambourne at Birmingham University. The course requires students to do a piece of original research or write an extended paper on a topic of their own choice arising out of their academic and practical work. The chapter following is the paper which he submitted in August 1968.

What has been attempted here is to look at some of the general anxieties that may be encountered in a psychiatric hospital; to see how these and others have helped to shape the defence system within a traditional set-up; and how a therapeutic community has tried to deal with the failure in communication and learning that such set-ups resulted in. The extent to which the new approaches with their flattened hierarchies have overcome these failures, and the problems they have had to face in their turn are also looked at. In more detail there is an examination of the presence of formal elements in the staff patterns and the possible tensions this arouses within a culture that seeks to flatten the staff hierarchy. The role of the doctor is given special consideration as one that has to face to a marked degree the problem of authority. This section is introduced by some remarks about the Buberian approach which I found exciting at this time and which I feel provides some valuable insights pertinent to the role of the therapist. In conclusion there is a brief look at patterns of leadership in the community, especially those of patients.

I should like to add one point in the hope that it might encourage someone to do something I had intended but have been unable to do. The therapeutic community might be a valuable model for comparison with the community of the local church as it tries to break away from past traditions of structure and hierarchy. There would be many lessons that it could offer and one would hope that a Christian community could also offer some insights in return. But at any rate in the matter of authority the two would have not dissimilar problems to face. For example, one only has to think about the problem of role-blurring and uncertainty as it affects the psychiatrist and clergyman.

Although some general comments on therapeutic communities are made they should be read in the light of the fact that I have direct experience at any depth of only one such community and have had to rely on published accounts of others for my wider knowledge. Unless explicitly stated to the contrary the detailed examples are in fact based upon my acquaintance with the John Conolly Hospital (JC) in Birmingham. In fairness to those who work and have been patients at the hospital I make it clear that my comments are based on very personal impressions. In the language of the Conolly, what follows is what 'I feel' about the problem of anxiety and authority in the therapeutic community. I am very grateful to them all at the hospital for the help they have given me and the very enjoyable time I had working there.

A. ANXIETY AND THE HOSPITAL

There is a witticism that one always comes across somewhere in contact with therapeutic communities. Someone at some point will jokingly tell you: 'In this place you can't tell the staff from the patients'. One has learnt of course to see jokes as a serious matter, even while smiling.[1] Topics under a social taboo may well appear in clownish disguise – and so too do our anxieties. It is therefore interesting to note that since it is the staff as much as the patients who are likely to make the comment (especially to a visitor), some sort of anxiety appears to be a fairly common feature in such communities. The precise nature of this anxiety is of course a very complex matter, but the more obvious aspects can provide a point of departure for what this paper is attempting to look at.

The 'madhouse fantasy'

Revans has made the general statement that 'the hospital is an

organism characterized by anxiety'.[2] Breaking this down a bit it
would be possible to see focal clusters of anxiety typical for particular
types of hospitals. Thus in the general hospital death, infection (with
its quasi-moral overtones of evil pollution) and physical contact
would be part of the characteristic focus. In a maternity hospital
anxiety might centre more upon fears of child abnormality, parental
responsibility, sex and reproductive roles. In mental hospitals it is
more likely to be violence, stigma, chronicity and the nature of sanity.

While in practice the use of drug therapy has meant that the
modern psychiatric hospitals are not characterized by the overt
expression of violence and the need for its control in the crudely
physical way of the old strait-jacket and padded cell, nevertheless the
popular image of the 'mad' is still heavily coloured by ideas of the
violently aggressive. Sensational journalism tends to reinforce this
with its reporting of hospital escapes and its description of a criminal
such as Frank Mitchell as the 'Mad axe-man'. Personal as well as
social fears about man's aggressive instincts find a useful scapegoat
in the mentally ill and a Western middle-class Christian heritage
with its emphasis on meekness as compliance and with no theology
of aggression, has only added to the general situation. It cannot be
denied, of course, that there are violent people in mental hospitals
and occasions of physical violence do still occur *in spite* of the use of
tranquillizers (or as David Cooper would say, *because* of the use of
tranquillizers, which can be used as the agents of 'violent' restraint
of a chemical as against the older, physical form).[3] Thus a factual
element becomes the fixing point of a whole burden of anxious
elaboration. And the manner in which the hospital deals with its
anxiety here is one indication of the general ideology and atmosphere
of the hospital. Staff and patients, especially the paranoid and the
neurotic, will find such occasions highly anxiety-provoking, in-
vesting them with their own unresolved feelings towards their own
aggressive impulses.

While in the public view the psychiatrist has a high status rating,
and although the public image of mental illness and mental hospitals
is improving, nevertheless the fact remains that it is widely felt that
mental illness and admittance to a mental hospital lowers one's
social prestige and bears a stigma. This seems to remain true even
with the increased number of voluntary patients. Fears of social,
employment, and family rejection often run high. Attempts to deal
with this both socially and by the individual are often little more

than covering-up tactics and denial. This can be seen, for example, in the way that words gradually take on 'stigma' associations and have to be replaced till they in turn become contaminated. Take, for example, the descriptions asylum, mental hospital, psychiatric hospital. The words may also reveal a change in the actual way patients are cared for, but not necessarily so. At the moment psychiatric hospital seems to be more acceptable than mental hospital. 'After all', a patient will say, 'I'm not mental', although he may well be pleased if he were told he was good at mental arithmetic. The stigma attitude probably has less telling effect upon the staff. Working at a mental hospital is probably seen by society as a particularly difficult task even within the general caring work of the medical and nursing professions and evidence of a special vocational sense. Society, however, is notoriously reluctant to give due monetary rewards for those considered to 'have a vocation', and within the medical sphere psychiatry remains something of a cinderella, especially in the British hospital service.

Chronicity, I would suggest, is a source of anxiety in the mental hospitals in some ways comparable (though obviously not equal) to that surrounding death in a general hospital. The presence of long-stay patients, especially those who show all the signs of institutionalization, is not only part of the fantasies surrounding mental hospitals but a source of anxiety both for patients and staff. It is true that present-day thinking and practice seek to find ways of avoiding the worst effects of institutionalization, and with new ventures and emphasis upon community care, stay in hospital is relatively reduced. But in fact at present, and probably for some time in the future too, hospital populations do and will contain chronic long-term patients. They are witness, as death is in the general hospital, of the limits of knowledge, practice and 'curing' possibilities within medical care. Thus for the patients, while doctors have something of the aura of the omniscient and the omnipotent about them, the chronic reveal the fallibility of those in whom one rests one's faith of help and health. For the staff they are reminders, in one sense healthy reminders, of areas of impotence. The depth of the anxiety that this arouses may be seen in the way some psychiatrists will welcome and put faith in new therapies – be they drugs, ECT, leucotomies, insulin or psychotherapy, some-times without due critical appraisal. The chance to 'do' something at last can be a powerful pressure and a relief to be grasped by staff for their own sake as much as for the patients. The history of the treatment of chronic schizophrenics would seem to show this.[4]

It could be said that what underlies many of the anxieties in a mental hospital is the anxiety about the nature of insanity, much as in general hospitals there is an underlying anxiety about illness. And obviously this point of view could be developed. But it seems to me that there is more bite to the question if we ask: What does it mean to be *sane*? What is the sanity a hospital is aiming for? Who are the sane? It is a part of and in some aspects parallel with the question that is increasingly being asked: What is health?

While medical shorthand no doubt requires an area of broadly agreed clinical description and terminology, the tendency is for this to feed lay fantasy with the impression of the clear distinction between the sane and the mad. A 'them and us' categorization helps to affirm a belief in one's own health more rigidly, and this is important where part of the 'stigma' anxiety connected with mental illness is seen in subconscious moralistic terms. That is, because mental illness is still quite largely seen in terms of failure (lack of will-power, lack of love, lack of control, etc.), it remains important that one should not be counted among the ill. But it is not only lay fantasy that plays a part here. The 'them/us' syndrome is not an uncommon feature in hospitals and among staff, however much sophistication of terminology may seek to give it respectability. In fact, of course, sanity/insanity are part of a continuum, not discreet modes of being and behaviour, and clinical categories are used with qualification and far from unanimous opinion. Is not this part of what the person who says, 'You can't tell the staff from the patients', is testifying to? For the staff, and especially for those working among the neurotic and on short-stay admittance units, it is clear, or should be, that there is a lot of 'them' in 'us' and no small part of 'us' in 'them'.

My experience at the JC would suggest to me that this 'them/us' approach is a frequently used defence mechanism, not only in staff/patient relations but also in staff/staff relations. The former may well take quite a subtle form since a 'democratic permissive' community makes open expression of this barrier defence more difficult. But I suspect that some of the 'descriptive' language for behaviour is given strong judgmental overtones which provide a mechanism for keeping patients, to some extent, 'in their place'. For example, the term 'anger' need not strictly in this setting be a 'bad' word.

The ability to express strong negative feelings can in fact have a positive value. Nevertheless, in almost all cases I have heard the word used of a patient it has had an almost 'moral' element and a tone of censure. So much so in one case that a patient gave as the reason for not talking in groups that he was always being told off for being angry. Clinical categories have the same latent potentials in them – as a defence and distancing of relations. There is the tendency at times for them to be used in this way, as indeed they are outside hospitals. David Martin, in a different context, says: 'A progressive wishing to discredit a particular person or viewpoint does not use the straightforward language of moral disapproval but employs the language of pathology.'[5]

There is also the danger of staff solidarity over against the patients. On the whole there was awareness of this and there were real efforts made not to present an unrealistically solid front, especially in the making and communicating of decisions. Nevertheless, occasions do occur that might need closer looking at. What, for example, are the implications of the statement: 'I thought the staff were working well together today in community', or the occasion when a patient had pressed the staff for a clear statement of general attitude that had in fact hit at several points of inter-staff tension and anxiety, but met with a total refusal to make reply, and the staff in the after-group dismissed the incident by saying: 'Wasn't he angry!' Among staff relations the them/us attitude appears in various ways. Jokingly, other doctors or nurses are said to be 'mad' or 'crazy'. In a situation where the hierarchy is flattened there is less opportunity for using a rank and status structure to provide a them/us generalization. But systems such as different teams, two nursing structures – administration and team, the distinction between night and day staff, all provide this means of positing blame and affirming oneself at the expense of others.

For the patient, the anxiety of sanity might well present itself in the form: 'What is being well, for me? What criteria will be used by those with the power (the staff) to decide my wellness? My way of being me does not seem so very different from the way they are they, so why is it me who is reckoned to be ill?' In those precise forms I doubt if such questions are asked, but they seem to lie behind some things that are said by patients.

What I have called the 'madhouse fantasy' would seem to me to be part of the general area of anxiety likely to be shared by any mental hospital. What would be distinctive in one place as against another would be the way in which these anxieties were dealt with or warded off, and that we will deal with a little later. The therapeutic communities share these with other forms of institutional care but may find certain aspects more pressing than they would and others easier to deal with.

Uncertainty of roles

Here we come much more clearly into the specific realm of the communities, for although role anxiety does exist in the more traditional psychiatric hospitals, the firmer structuring of their social systems and hierarchies act as a clearer defence against it.

H. H. Perlman, in a useful discussion of the role concept in social case-work, describes the meaning of 'role' in these terms: 'our individual, personal ways of communicating are for the most part contained within, coloured by and fashioned by certain over-all socially determined, and organized patterns of expected behaviour. These patterns of expected behaviour – and by "behaviour" we mean not only what is done but also the accompanying effects – are called "roles". Social roles mark out what a person in a given social position and situation is expected to be, act like, and to feel like and what the other(s) in relation to him are expected to be, to act like and to feel like.'[6]

In our normal social intercourse we gradually learn roles appropriate for everyday circumstances. It would be possible to see child education and development in terms of socialization – that is the acquisition of appropriate role sets, and the family as the fundamental socializing instrument or medium. Goode says: 'the family is the fundamental instrumental foundation of the larger social structure, and . . . all other institutions depend on its contributions. The role behaviour that is learned within the family becomes the model or prototype for role behaviour required in other segments of the society.'[7,8] But clearly this process is continual, and with society more mobile the need for adapting behaviour to new situations is increasing. New social situations carry with them new exciting possibilities, of course, but also anxiety since one is uncertain about behaviour expectations appropriate for the new situation. Often there will be some transfer of learning from past experience, and some element of generalization is usually possible, but the new elements are what are likely to trouble us. For example, a schoolboy will have learnt his role as pupil *vis-à-vis* the role of teacher and the role of other pupils. On leaving school and entering university he enters a new social situation which contains something of the old elements but also demands role-adaptation as well. If he goes straight into a job, then the adaptation is wider and the anxiety relatively greater.

Similarly, on being admitted to hospital one enters a new social situation. The world of the hospital enjoys its own social system and structure and its own sub-culture. Within it there are role stratifications, ideologies, sanctions, and behaviour expectations. Whether as staff or as patient one is expected to learn a role. In general terms there is probably some preparation for this. Even before entering we have some broad ideas of what is likely to be expected, though this may well contain a high level of fantasy. There will be some notion of what a patient is expected to do or not do, built up in part at least on previous doctor/patient relations. But in detail there often remains a great deal to be learnt, as is pointed out by Revans.[9]

The model for hospitalization that most people have revolves round the general hospital with its recumbent patient presenting his set of symptoms and a hierarchy of medical/nursing personnel doing things. At the pinnacle is the doctor before whom all bow. This model has, by and large, been adopted in psychiatric hospitals and thus broadly conforms to expectations. And one of the most basic expectations is the fundamental distinction between staff and patients. But development of therapeutic communities, units and 'anti-hospitals' clearly shows that there has been dissatisfaction with this general model when it comes to the institutional care of the mentally ill. Within these new structures, new social systems and new behaviour expectancies have developed. The old role-models have been modified, sometimes quite drastically, and as our joke reveals, one of the basic areas of change has been that of patient/staff role distinction. If what has been said up till now is in any way valid it would suggest that since the therapeutic community does not conform to the popular expectation of what it means to be in a hospital, the degree of role-learning required is greater and is to some extent at odds with what might be called role-preparation, which is based on individual expectation of what a hospital involves and the general model society has of hospital care.

As an attempt to allay some of the anxieties that could arise from this, some communities send out introductory letters to patients soon to be admitted giving a brief picture of what can be expected.[10] In JC a booklet is given to each new patient on admission giving brief information about the main hospital activities and its general approach.

More detailed examination of role uncertainty and its implications will appear in the succeeding sections.

B. ANXIETY AND THE HIERARCHY

The development of the hierarchical, autocratic set-up in a hospital can be traced in part to the two main lines of nursing care, namely the military and the religious, and also in part to an unconscious or subconscious systematizing of defences against the anxieties pervading hospital care. For a discussion of this and the short-comings of such systems as studied in a general teaching hospital, see I. Menzies: 'A Case-study in the Functioning of Social Systems as a Defence against Anxiety.'[11] While due caution should be shown in transferring her findings into the world of the mental hospital, nevertheless it would appear that sufficient areas of common anxiety and structure patterns can be found for our present purposes.

Miss Menzies argues that: 'The work situation arouses very strong and mixed feelings in the nurse: pity, compassion and love; guilt and anxiety; hatred and resentment of the patients who arouse these strong feelings; envy of the care given to the patient.'

Within this objective situation there are, she suggests, strong re-semblances to fantasy situations that can be traced back to infancy. Using a Kleinian approach she sees here the primitive conflict and tension between the libido and aggressive forces in the individual with the anxiety of an uncontrolled aggression especially powerful. Because of the closeness between the real and the fantasy situation in hospital work, the nurse 'is at considerable risk of being flooded by intense and unmanageable anxiety'. The level of anxiety in a hospital, however, cannot be accounted for purely from this factor and so Miss Menzies studied what she calls the 'socially structured defence mechanism' of the hospital set-up. 'A social defence system develops over time as the result of collusive interaction and agreement, often unconscious, between members of the organization as to what form it shall take. The socially structured defence mechanisms then tend to become an aspect of external reality with which old and new members of the institution must come to terms.'

As some of the elements of this system she mentions: splitting up of the nurse/patient relationship by a system of task lists; de-personalization, categorism and denial of the significance of the individual; detachment and denial of feelings; attempt to eliminate decisions by ritual task performance; the reduction of the impact of responsibility by delegation to superiors. By this system anxiety is only faced by avoidance. 'Little attempt is made positively to help the individual confront the anxiety-evoking experience and, by doing so, to develop her capacity to tolerate and deal more effectively with the anxiety.' The defences in fact are working at a primitive and not mature level and so tend towards the evasion of anxiety rather than its true modification and reduction. But with all this there goes a very strong resistance to any form of radical change, so that while nurses experience deep anxiety and may even be able to see that the set-up aggravates the situation, the deep fear of change confirms the *status quo*. At breaking point the individual and not the system goes – hence high turnovers in staff.

Out of the large numbers of very important details that this study revealed, it is possible, I think, to extract two lines of general thought: the pattern of hierarchy and its relation to communication.

In this section an attempt will be made to see in what ways the therapeutic communities have reacted against these aspects of the traditional hospital system and what problems arise out of their own system.

The traditional hierarchy

The social system of the traditional hospital is based upon a firm pyramid structure with the superintendent at the top and nursing assistants and training nurses arrayed along the bottom. As a sort of sub-strata there would be the domestics, porters and so on. Within the pyramid clear lines of stratification could be drawn with firm lines between various grades, e.g. the very firm one between the medical and nursing staff, and another one between the trained and untrained nurses. Patients are not part of this structure, but have a clearly defined role within the total hospital system. At simplest they are the receivers of the healing care of the hospital, the ones to be cured or guarded. It is largely a passive, dependent role. It is a matter of debate whether or not the role of the patient is the focus of the *raison d'être* of a hospital. While it might be assumed that every hospital is there primarily for the sake of its patients, the facts do not always seem to bear this out. In some of the larger teaching and research hospitals it appears to some people that the patient is there in fact for the sake of the hospital. For example, N. Exchaquet, President of the Swiss Association of Graduate Nurses, has said: 'The evolution of the hospital by producing a number of pre-occupations other than the patient in its very heart has made of him an article of popular consumption, in fact, indispensable in respect of the scientific, teaching, technical and economic objectives of the establishment.'[12]

Within this autocratic system authority lies with those above one in the structure and deference is expected to that authority or status. Individual responsibility and initiative are reduced, especially in the lower strata, to a task performance set at a general level for each particular status. The tendency is for the individual to be hidden by the rank – objectified in the differences made in the uniforms and terms of address, and worked out in a task system. Throughout the hierarchy there is a tendency to see those above as imposing an unnecessarily strict supervision and to see those below as irresponsible and to treat them as such. Miss Menzies says of this, that it reveals 'a collusive system of denial, splitting and projection that is culturally acceptable to, indeed culturally required of, nurses. . . . Each nurse tends to split off aspects of herself from her conscious personality and to project them into other nurses. Her irresponsible impulses, which she fears she cannot control, are attributed to her juniors. Her painfully severe attitude to these impulses and burdensome sense of responsibility are attributed to her seniors. Consequently, she identifies juniors with the irresponsible self and treats them with the severity that self is felt to deserve. Similarly, she identifies seniors with her own harsh disciplinary attitude to her irresponsible self. There is psychic truth in the assertion that juniors are irresponsible and seniors harsh disciplinarians. These are the roles assigned to them. There is also objective truth, since people act objectively on the psychic roles assigned them.'[13] The system thus establishes itself and persists out of a collusive acceptance and exertion of authoritarian rule, although at the same time it gives rise to repeated expressions of dissatisfaction and complaint. Yet the system itself gives no legitimate way of registering the complaint. The reality of the tensions and anxieties is endured for fear of the possibly greater initial pain that might bring restoration.[14] This system, therefore, has the potentials within it of the very type of covert staff tensions which, in Stanton and Schwarz's hypothesis, are found out in the overt disturbances of patients.[15]

Another area in which this system frequently gives rise to frustration and anxiety is that of communication. Something of the connection between the lines of thought can be seen in this comment from the introduction to *Standards for Morale*: 'In our view, any lack of sympathy occasionally displayed by those in authority does not so much derive from defects in their personalities as from the anxiety based on lack of understanding, upon imperfect information, or even upon the misconception of their professional roles. These in turn derive from inadequate communication, which is both cause and product of unfavourable attitudes.'[16] 'Uncertainty is magnified by communication failure. . . . A regenerative process may start: anxiety, uncertainty, communication blockage, *anxiety uncertainty*, *communication blockage*. ANXIETY, UNCERTAINTY, COMMUNICATION BLOCKAGE.'[17] Revans goes on to say that along with this there goes the need to learn, so as to relieve the anxiety, etc., but because of the vicious circle the very processes of learning are themselves blocked. And this is particularly true for those on the lower rungs of the hierarchy ladder. He found that lines of information ran vertically upwards, always towards those in authority, to senior staff that they may be fully informed, free of doubt. In fact, that they may learn. No such system was available to those along the lower orders – and that includes patients – helping them in their adjustment to hospital life. In fact the traditional system is highly unsuited to assist in the learning processes of those in subordinate positions, 'and the extent to which it happens to be possible is the extent to which the hospital is, in this sense, unofficial, informal, unconventional'. 'Control systems to keep informed those who are in charge are not enough; the stoker in the engine room no less than the captain on the bridge needs to understand what is going on. We must give more thought than we have in the past to the problems thrown up by change and emergency at all levels and this demands that many of those in authority shall have a new perception of their relations, both formal and informal, to their subordinates.'[18]

We have looked at the traditional hierarchy of staff structures in terms of two closely linked ideas – as a defence system against anxiety and as a communication system in the process of learning, or what we earlier called adaptation. In both these areas we have found evidence that the system has some serious shortcomings. Perhaps this is a suitable point to note that we have not been attempting a systematic assessment of the orthodox system. Had we done so the over-all impression may not have been so negative. Clearly it is much easier to present a one-sided picture in order to push home a criticism, but it is necessary to remember that the total truth may be more complicated. This is said, not because I feel the points made are invalid but because I am conscious that they are selected points and it is necessary to be aware of the dangers of selection.

Having made that qualification, however, I want to go on now to see how far changes in the formal structure of the hierarchy go towards meeting the shortcomings.

The flattening of the hierarchy

To see the flattening of the hierarchy within the therapeutic communities as merely a reaction against the traditional forms would be to over-simplify the history of the development of such communities. The questioning of the old structures is at least partly a consequence of the thinking that has sprung from their development and not merely a causal factor. And in any case, the new structures are the product of experiment, of the working through of tensions, and of the meeting of new demands over a number of years and in many different places. Just as a picture of the traditional system can only be a very general one modified in its details and effectiveness with each individual place, so too the newer patterns vary with each community. General lines may be visible but there is no master blue-print to which each community refers and tries to copy *in toto*.

Thus, while the work and ideas of a man like Maxwell Jones have been seminal for much in this area in this country, and although for many he is seen to be something of the prophet (and high priest) for the 'movement', individual hospitals show a healthy and necessary divergence from patterns established, for example, at the Henderson or Dingleton. Maxwell Jones himself has said: 'The fact is, of course, that there is, as yet, no one model of a therapeutic community and all that is intended is that it should mobilize the interest, skills and enthusiasms of staff and patients and give them sufficient freedom of action to create their own optimal treatment and living

conditions. In such circumstances, what will emerge will be characteristic for the particular group and may have little in common with
other therapeutic communities.'[19] Nevertheless, with due caution, it
is possible to make some generalizations.

The flattening of hierarchy and the freeing of communication
are aspects of the same movement and, like a pair of horses har-
nessed together, depend upon the efforts of each other. They are
part of a dynamic, giving it expression and driving force, but
without each other will only lead to upsetting the cart. It would not
be possible to encourage the relaxing of strict autocratic rule and the
introduction of a 'flatter' or less rigid hierarchy, if at the same time
there were not the openness throughout the system to free lines of
communication and lay one self open to the demands that this will
make. Clearly the imposition of what purports to be less authoritarian is a practical contradiction. It is rather like saying that everyone
can do what they like as long as they do what I tell them to do and
like it. There is the danger of giving assent to a 'good idea' without
actually risking its being put into real practice. This can be seen, I
suspect, in some of the claims in hospitals that 'here we work as a
team' while in practice it works more like a régime. What makes a
team real is not the insistence upon it as a concept but the atmosphere
between the members, its morale: not the law which says 'Thou shalt
be a team' but the spirit that makes it a living possibility. And this
means that there has to be the freedom to speak out, to ask why
and to query those above one in the formal structure as well as those
below.

But the freeing of communication is equally an unrealized ideal
if it does not go with a relaxing of the authority structure. To give
lip service to an openness of attitude and yet insist upon one's own
status position and the deference to be shown to it, is to ask for a
too easy salvation from the problems caused by blocked communications. To free communication means meeting people beyond
the confines of rank with a willingness to have demands made upon
one and the strength to face criticism from lower as well as higher
ranks. As Revans says: 'Those within the hospital, or at least a
majority of them, must perceive that their subordinates, in order
to learn, must be permitted to make unprogrammed demands upon
their supervisors. These demands, moreover, may be expected to
disturb or even threaten; they may come at times inconvenient to
the senior; they may question, even if unintentionally, the authority,

knowledge, judgment or values of the senior; they may bring to the senior facts or interpretations of facts that he or she would prefer not to recognize; they may suggest a need for change in the senior, change that might be not merely difficult but painful.'[20]

Christianity has always been aware of the cost of 'salvation', and psychiatry too knows that pain is involved in the process of developing emotional and relational maturity and health. Flattening a hierarchy and freeing communication are similarly no cheap means of grace by which the anxieties and tensions we saw evident in the traditional set-up can be dealt with. The opposite is perhaps nearer the truth. The traditional way was a method of retreat from anxiety without ever being a satisfactory way of learning how it might be reduced. But the new structures require that tension and anxiety be faced while at the same time providing, at best, the support and help which make the facing of anxiety a joint and not merely a solitary affair.

But how does all this work out in practice? The flattening of a hierarchy clearly does not mean that the hierarchy disappears. But what it does mean is that there is a breaking down of barrier lines that typified the pyramid structure so that movement of communication and relationship is on quite a new direction and plane. This might be represented in a number of different ways: it is more direct, more horizontal than vertical; dialogical rather than monological.

It is more direct, both in the sense that communication and relationship are not mediated so often through layers of hierarchy, and also in the sense that with greater openness there is a legitimate 'system' for registering forthright feelings to those involved, no matter where they stand within the hierarchy. Associated with this is the idea of 'confrontation' by which any member of the community (patients as well as staff) can be faced with their behaviour, decisions, attitudes, etc., not in the atmosphere of a trial but rather as a learning situation whereby feelings of other members can be brought out and the reality of the total situation examined. It is perhaps unfortunate that 'confrontation' tends to take on bad associations so that it is seen to be a crisis event when there is something pretty obviously wrong either in actions or, for example, inter-staff relations, and the positive value of confrontation as a way to learn tends to get lost. It is also unfortunate that direct expression of feelings most often means the expression of rather negative feelings. It is much rarer for there to be mention of approval at the way a nurse, doctor or patient acted in a certain situation, than for querying of attitudes and actions. But this possibility of open and direct approach can be a way of reducing 'locker room' back-biting and the frustration of having no accepted way to make a face-to-face comment of either approval or disapproval. This is most obvious in the relations between the members of those parts of the hierarchy traditionally furthest apart.

The new lines of movement are more horizontal than vertical. In discussing Revans' point about communication we noted that the system of information in a traditional set-up was authority-organized for the sake of those in authority and hence tended to be a one-way process: information travelling upward and orders descending from rank to rank. The problem for the subordinate ranks was the Why of the command, both the way it was to fit in with the over-all picture and what to do if one wanted to query it. With greater directness of approach between ranks, however, and without lines of intermediary ranks between top and bottom, the line of movement is more as between peers and hence horizontal. In practice this is more complex than it may have sounded. The nursing assistant may have equal right to express her opinion and ask for information as does the doctor, but there are senses in which they are not (or at least do not 'feel') equal. Between these opposite ends of the formal hierarchy there are clear differences in knowledge and role which cannot help affecting the relationship, but in the middle ranks, e.g. SEN and SRN, the role distinction is even less clear. At best this means that there are potentials for conflict just because the roles have become blurred and it is no longer accepted practice to retreat into a status rank in order to relieve the possible anxieties of role uncertainty. Such anxiety may well be increased under the flattened hierarchy system, for within the community there are few tasks that cannot be interchanged among the various levels of staff. As a charge nurse recently commented, 'We should advertise for a therapist who will also do domestic duty.' The task list method which links status with a clear function area no longer holds where 'all' are considered therapists. Certain administrative functions may well be the prerogative of sisters or charge nurses but in any given situation the level of responsibility and initiative required of an individual may bear little relation to the formal rank he or she enjoys. For example, a domestic member of staff may well be the

only staff member in a group, and in that situation she has a therapeutic responsibility which all the staff share (and in a sense all
patients as well).

The new method of communication will be dialogical and not
monological. In simple form the distinction might be seen in the
difference between 'talking with' and 'speaking to or at', or in the
use of 'we' rather than 'you'. Something of this might be seen by
comparing the two sermons by Father Paneloux in *The Plague*. Of
the second the narrator says: 'He spoke in a gentler, more thoughtful
tone than on the previous occasion, and several times was noticed
to be stumbling over his words.' A yet more noteworthy change was
that instead of saying 'You' he now said 'We'.[21] Or one might think
of the difference between the lecture and the seminar. Both are forms
of human communication, but in dialogue we are expressing and
discovering what it is to be more truly human together. In dialogue
we are at risk, in monologue we have not allowed ourselves to become
vulnerable. To open communications and lay aside the defensive
barriers of rank is to open the way to vulnerability but also to the
opportunity to learn and hence to grow. The risks of living dialogi-
cally have already been implied and the temptation to retreat from
this form of relationship are continual. In a therapeutic community
that form of monologue that is based on 'pulling rank' is less easy
to get away with because the general culture is against it, but subtle
sophistications of the monologue appear often enough, especially
at times of special anxiety, e.g. at times of more than usual dis-
turbance among patients, or when individual staff members are at
odds with each other, or when major changes in organization are in
the offing.

Those who work in a therapeutic community would no doubt see
these as ideals that are only relatively put into practice. The problem
of confrontation has already been mentioned. There is often resistance to this method of learning and communication. The ideology
of the place works towards facilitating the expression of feelings,
but in other ways it may be found that the community culture
makes communication more difficult. This is particularly noticeable
in the communication of decisions. As we shall see later, when
looking more specifically at authority, there are problems anyway
in the making of decisions, and the ambivalence that surrounds that
process spills over into the process of communicating them. Ideally,
the various systems of feedback that communities adopt ensure that

information from throughout the community and throughout the day can be made available to any individual. In practice, however, the volume of information is such that there is often a confusion between the trivial and the significant. Further, because of the verbal nature of the material and because it is not always possible for the person who needs the relevant information to be on the spot when the feedback is given, there develops a very informal and at times haphazard system of hearsay and grapevine. Moreover, the reluctance of those in authority to provide answers in group meetings with patients may well have a therapeutic purpose, but there is the danger that direct information answers come to be seen as essentially bad in themselves and staff are left to gauge group feelings in a staff meeting over a matter that required a clear answer. For example: a sudden and marked increase in the number of bed patients had put real strains on the nursing staff. There was therefore some pressure upon the medical staff to review the need of some of the patients to be kept in bed. Some confusion had been experienced over one of these patients as to whether or not he should be allowed up, and on one day he had apparently spent the time being put to bed by one nurse and being got up again by another. A clear directive was requested of the doctor in charge of the patient as to what he wanted done. This was made at a staff meeting. After a quarter of an hour of varied comments and considerable silence the meeting closed with there still being no answer to the question. When tackled again the doctor said the nurse had had her answer in the group – which only added confusion and frustration to the situation.

The difficulty here is that because there was no clear answer (difficult as it may have been to give one) the nurse acts on a level of guesswork on her own opinion which in the course of events may or may not be in accordance with the wishes of the doctor. The crunch comes if the 'wrong' thing is done, which is very easily possible since each nurse in the group may have 'read' the answer of the group differently.

The practical implications of the flattened hierarchy can be seen almost immediately one enters a therapeutic community. For a start there is the lack of uniform, which is perhaps the most obvious outward symbol of the hierarchy structure in the traditional hospital. The difference this makes to initial anxieties is perhaps telling. The array of different uniforms in a traditional hospital sets up a cluster of anxieties which would probably include the fear of consequences of one's ignorance through the possibility of calling matron 'nurse' and the orderly 'sister'. One has recognized that there is a clear social structure present within which there will be clear roles and appropriate forms of address and behaviour, but the anxiety occurs because one has not yet learnt to distinguish the ranks and thus the fear of inappropriate behaviour. But on entering the therapeutic community the initial anxiety is more confused. There is the un-expectedness and a fear of a wider ignorance, not merely how 'they' rank themselves but which 'they' in fact are. We are with our initial joke again. Although this initial confusion may well therefore be greater, since all, except doctors, are known by Christian names and the staff do not array themselves in terms of rank, the confusion resolves itself into something more like realistic basis for relationship. Occasionally one hears from both staff and patients the desire that staff should wear uniforms. It is possible to make out quite a reason-able case for this, but behind it all one suspects that there is a high level of anxiety, role uncertainty and a desire to be able to meet on the level of pre-structured relationship. A uniform, after all, provides a level of defence by means of a degree of anonymity and generaliza-tion. With a stethoscope round his neck this man is doctor and not merely Mr Jones. A role structure is established immediately. The sister's blue uniform and starched cap establishes a type of authority which goes with the rank regardless, at the outset, of the person inside the uniform. They are the sacramental vestments of the hospital.

What goes on in the frequent staff meetings and after groups is a more telling evidence of the authenticity of the flattened hierarchy, how far it is something more than a concept. The freedom of inter-change and expression of real feelings can be on very different levels, and while the initial break with a traditional system and the very existence of such groups makes a new level of communication and relationship possible, it probably takes a community staff a long time to learn how to use the new possibilities with real effectiveness. And even once established it is never assured in a situation that is by necessity on-going and changing. New pressures and anxieties, change of staff and experiment with new approaches mean an ever fluid situation. And this means constant adaptation and learning. The danger of a long-established community is that, just as in the traditional set-up, systems become stereotyped to meet the cultural needs and provide defences. The hope is that with openness and less emphasis upon the formal structures there is a better awareness of these dangers and a greater readiness to meet the difficulties. But it is essential that this be a matter faced by the group in support of individuals. Inadequate as we have seen the old defence system to be, it nevertheless did provide some sort of defence. Under this more flexible open system the inadequacies are only made good if realistic and adequate support in the face of anxieties and confusion over role is provided. 'Therapy', after all, is not a matter of stripping away all defences and leaving the personality naked, but the giving of help by which the individual may develop mature defences and a stronger personality.

I said earlier that flattening of the hierarchy does not mean that the hierarchy disappears, and before concluding this section it is necessary to say something of the continuing place of the formal hierarchy in the therapeutic community and some of the problems that this raises.

Not only does the formal hierarchy provide a fairly clear role picture, it also provides a structure of authority and responsibility. It is not sufficient to be aware merely of its shortcomings. The enunciation of decisions and commands that cannot be questioned can at worst become a form of authoritarian dictatorship, stunting initiative and responsibility. But that form of society which continually fails to come to decisions, where decisions are both required and necessary, reveals an irresponsibility that verges on anarchy. Democracy attempts to meet this by the election of representatives and the delegation of authority into their hands while the elective body retains ultimate authority and power in the strength of the vote. Although therapeutic communities sometimes use the word democracy to describe its social system, it is clear that the word is being used in a special way. 'In the Unit', says Rapaport of the Belmont Unit, 'the authority, or legitimated power, is formally assigned to the staff, who also hold formal responsibility. The staff is a numerical minority which informally shares its authority and responsibility with others in the Unit because of its ideology of democratization. One major problem here is that authority and responsibility tend to be diffused differentially. Many people are eager to accept authority without being willing to take the responsibility that may go with it. Since in the Unit both attributes remain formally with the staff, they are left with the problem of having frequently to accept responsibility for the disruptive use of power which they have informally vested in the patients'.[22]

We shall have to return to this question of authority and responsibility diffusion, but for the moment it is sufficient to say that the same sort of problem arises within the staff situation as well. Certain authority and responsibility is vested in the holders of certain positions according to rank. But with the arrangement by which many decisions are presented to groups to make and indeed authority given to individuals who do not also have the responsibility, confusion and tensions can and do arise. For example, a group together with a nurse may come to the decision that a patient should be allowed to drive his car. But the responsibility for that person's safety and public safety is not in the hands of the nurse or the patients but with the doctor. And the position is further complicated by the requirements of an external authority, the law.

Another aspect can be seen in this example. The nursing staff were divided between those on administrative nursing and those allocated to the doctors' teams. A patient in team A had stripped her bed and left the clothes strewn over the floor and the bed on its side. The sister in charge of the admin. nurses asked the SEN from the team to help remake the bed. The SEN felt this was not helpful to the patient and that she should remake it herself. The SEN was acting on the unspoken authority of the team. The sister, however, insisted with the weight of status that the bed be made. In a community where direct orders are rare rather than frequent it becomes harder to obey them even when it is required by the situation, which it probably was not in this case. At conflict here were not only formal and informal authority but approaches to 'therapy' and ward administration, as well as tensions existing between admin. and team nurses. Ideally the suggested solution would have been for the SEN to help with the bed and then confront the sister with the decision in terms of therapy and their joint feelings.

The problem with hierarchy is that formally it exists and yet with reduced significance, and that it is in some ways replaced by a fluctuating informal hierarchy. The formal aspects of it are apparent in certain functions, e.g. sisters or charge nurses make out supply requisitions, duty lists and write reports. It is also seen in terms of pay of course. It is partly obliterated by Christian names and large areas of function and role interchange – even extended to some areas across the medical/nursing line.

Informally the hierarchy is maintained by such things as the use of bleeps, the holders of drug keys, the use of an office, and those who do and do not call the consultants by their Christian names. In terms of the day-to-day working the balance between the formal and informal aspects operates sufficiently smoothly, but in times of stress or crisis the pressures are largely upon an increase in the formal aspects of an authority structure, although these are the very times when the openness of a freer informality are especially needed. In part this is the problem of running a community according to its self-developed system and culture and yet also being part of a wider structure controlling the staffing finances and status. It means that at times the two systems come into conflict, or at least tension, and the wider system provides some degree of escape from the anxieties furnished by the local situation. This, of course, has much broader implications than merely in the matter of staffing and staff relations, and opens up the whole question of the relationship of the community and its sub-culture to the rest of society, the purposes of therapy and its relation with rehabilitation. These have been studied in considerable detail in the research already referred to by Rapaport at the Belmont Unit.

What I want to stress here, however, is that as under a strictly formal structure informal sub-structures nevertheless develop, often with strong practical implications, so too where the emphasis is more on the side of the informal there remain formal elements which still exert a practical influence. In either set-up the danger is tacitly to ignore that element that runs counter to the major emphasis, failing to take it sufficiently into account. Since systems give expression to ideologies it requires maturity in the society to give open recognition to these 'heretical' elements. But reality requires that these layers are recognized and the relationship between the two openly considered so that the positive values can be made use of. Unless this is done the 'non-U' elements are a source of tension and guilt and the subconscious focus for grievance. In the case of the conflict between the SEN and the sister just referred to, for example, one of the underlying tensions not brought out at the time but expressed in a different context and general discussion, was the tension in a relationship between a nurse with less qualification yet with longer experience and informal authority over against the higher qualified but younger person with formal authority.

In this section we have looked at the staffing structures in both the traditional and community set-up, looking especially at the problem of anxiety and communication. Some of the problems that have been pointed out by Menzies and Revans arising from the rigid formal system can be seen to have at least potential answers in the more informal system found in the therapeutic community. But it would be quite false to conclude from this that a generalized pattern could be taken over from the communities and planted into each and every hospital. It is not the system or the lack of system that itself creates solutions, but the willingness of the individuals and the group to face the opportunities and the tensions in a learning way. Just as better communication cannot be guaranteed merely by the installation of more advanced technical equipment but needs the willingness and intention of the people involved to 'communicate' with each other, so too the establishment of staff groups does not guarantee better staff relations if there is not the willingness to face and express feelings and to learn from them in the supportive atmosphere provided by each for each. Nor should it be thought that communities have found all the answers. In many ways they are more likely to be the ones to admit that things are far from clear or successful. Learning for communities and groups is no less painful than it is for individuals, possibly more so. The problems of role uncertainty and of the relationship between given structures and the needs of the particular situation are more acute in the communities.

Each one has to struggle to its own solutions. This is pointed out by Revans: 'Our thesis is that such a community may be made whole only by itself, by those who work in it. There is no Ministry of Health prototype, no external example, no textbook model, no Platonic ideal on which it can be fashioned; there is no perfection to be brought about by administrative decree or departmental order alone; those who serve the hospital must perceive their own problems by their own lights and work out their solutions in their own ways.'[23]

C. AUTHORITY

I want to begin this section with quotations from two men of quite different backgrounds, speaking in quite different spheres of concern. Both of them testify to the widespread nature of the problem we are here concerned with and set the particulars of what is to be said in the necessary broader context. The first quotation appears in a book of collected lectures and writings of one of the prophets of the church's ecumenical endeavour, Albert H. van den Heuvel: 'Von Oppen has rightly said that the tension of this age is related to the fact that people recognize at the same time the fundamental equality of all people and the need for recognized authority. Authority, therefore, has to be fought for. . . . In practice this means that the wrong people seize it and enforce it by illegitimate means. Only a society that is structured in teams and partnership will be able to overcome the authority problem.'[24] And the second quotation is from the book by David H. Clark on Administrative Therapy: 'Western society during our life time, has seen so many shifts of attitude towards authority that we are all sensitive and easily made anxious on this account.'[25]

From van den Heuvel, I wish to pin-point three factors that seem to me to be relevant implications:

(i) Concern for the basic equality of individuals is not incompatible with the need for and expressions of authority.
(ii) Authority has legitimate as well as illegitimate modes of expression.
(iii) A social system built on partnership (a 'democracy' as the word is used in the therapeutic communities) should be the place for discovering solutions to the problem.

And David Clark's point, especially in the context of his study of the therapeutic milieu, provides something of a clue to why it is that even in a partnership society there is no easy solution to the problem. There is a sensitiveness that is all too conscious of the dangers of assertive authority and the fight for its power, and therefore is uneasy with any exercise of authority lest it should fall into the traps of authoritarianism. And yet because the exercise of authority of some sort seems to be required by a social system and in the interchange of human relations, it cannot be banished from the scene. The anxiety takes root in the confusion of those who have to find the narrow way between domination and abdication and in the guilty feeling of having stepped to one side or the other. In the course of this section we shall be looking in some detail at how this affects some of the various roles in a community, but first of all we shall be concerned with the broader issues of the nature of authority.

Authentic authority

We are here taking up an aspect of the second point of van den Heuvel. His terminology was legal and in sociology this is the terminology usually employed in a discussion of authority. The verb that springs to mind in the use of this terminology is that of 'having'– the position, status and power one *has*, and it would seem to present a model of structures of control backed up by a legalistic sanctioning system.

While this aspect of authority is not absent in the therapeutic community, it is an aspect that tends to be played down. Instead, the emphasis seems to be on authority in terms of what is authentic. Here the verb is 'being' – not so much what one *has* as what one *is*. The important thing is not the structures which provide a pre-shaped package in which people play out their roles already provided, but rather an open situation shared by all involved and out of which the role-structures evolve in the relationship of being together. One is repeatedly hearing the phrase 'unstructured groups' which I take to mean, not only does the group have no pre-determined plan of operation or agenda but that also the roles of each member and the 'abode' of authority is not pre-set either. Thus, far from imposing an already established authority structure, there are attempts made to break down the structures to allow the emergence of what is real or authentic in the given particular situation. The 'unstructured group' therefore might be said to represent not only a mode of therapy but also the model for a community's attitude to authority.

If one were to try and generalize about the two approaches we have been discussing, it would be possible to set up a series of word pairs: juridical, existential; official, personal; pre-structured, open; abstracted, *in situ*; generalized, particular; form, process; etc. Underlying all this there seems to be a divergence in the way of looking at things as old as the hills or at least as old as classical Greek philosophy, represented by the twin tradition of Plato and Aristotle. As a crude generalization it might be said that the one concentrates on the archetypal Ideal on whose pattern the particular is constructed, and the other emphasizes the emergence of the particular reality in the process of growth. The one is the building of a machine from the given plans, the other is the growth of an organism from the given 'material'.[26]

It is possible to see these two lines of approach worked out in almost all spheres of thought and activity – philosophy, theology education, psychology, art, etc., but although logically they are incompatible they are often held together in order to account for the fullness of the data to be dealt with (see the doctrine of complementarity). We should therefore be rightly cautious in giving to either total or exclusive adherence. In terms of our own topic this means that authority is neither solely a matter of the established structures nor is it purely a matter of what emerges in the particular shared situation of a given moment. Or to put it another way, human relations are neither the playing out of rigidly determined role-patterns unmodified by the actual interplay of the actual persons involved, nor are they merely the spontaneous meeting together of individuals unaffected by the experience and roles brought with them from the past and from the wider situation.

There is nothing very startling about this, of course, unless one insists upon a rigid conformity on the one hand or an existential extremism on the other. The differences occur in the degree to which one side or the other is given major expression – whether in the 'doing' of relationships the emphasis is upon 'having' or 'being' authority. The problem lies in the finding of a mode of 'doing' which is neither imposition nor abdication. If the danger of the orthodox, traditional hospital set-up has been to exercise authority as imposition, then the temptation of the radical community is to react with abdication.

David Cooper has gone so far as to say that distinguishing between authentic and inauthentic authority is the central problem of the psychiatric hospital, and he goes on to describe authentic leadership in this way: 'Perhaps the most central characteristic of authentic leadership is the relinquishing of the impulse to dominate others. Domination here means controlling the behaviour of others, where their behaviour represents for the leader projected elements of his own personality and experience. By domination of the others the leader produces from himself the illusion that his own internal organization is more perfectly ordered.'[27]

We have already seen from the study by Miss Menzies how the presence of anxiety builds up defence systems fed by personal fantasies, and how this affects relationships through the hierarchy. But it is not only the one who dominates who is seeking an orderliness that the situation within the self or in the social context belies. This is true also of those who are dominated, and for them

c

there is the illusion of order in the unquestioned obedience to the dominating command. The reciprocal nature of authority is frequently referred to by those writing on this topic. ' "Control" is, in fact, unavoidably mutual. To pretend that this mutuality of responsibility and power is not present in any group is illusion or delusion.'[28] 'The model system for the conventional institution is the delightfully landscaped cabbage patch. As cabbages live comfortably enough, at least until they go into the soup, many patients collude with the illusion of their keepers, and this interplay of illusion and collusion constitutes the basic social-fantasy system upon which the structure of the conventional institution is erected.'[29] 'Authority does not become effective except as the person towards whom it is exercised sanctions its use and acts in accord with the intention of the authority person.'[30] 'It is only if the client accepts the worker's authority that he will change the way the worker wants, whether the methods used are rational or authoritarian in form.'[31]

These last two quotations prompt me to make a slight digression for a moment. It would seem to me that in the more recent writings that appear in books and journals on the nature and practice of case-work, there is a new willingness to speak in positive terms about the place of authority. Thus, the opening words of Elliot Studt's article: 'A framework for study of the social worker's authority towards the client was not necessary when the profession was saying that casework could not be "done" from an authority position . . . but recently the profession has been noting that all social workers use authority in some way or other . . . If it is true that authority appears in all helping relationships then we should agree about what authority is.'[32]

A. W. Hunt, in the same volume, goes into the question of the *positive* value of enforced help as experienced in the probation service, helping to free the situation from the guilt that has no doubt been felt by many officers in trying to square client-determination, etc., with the pre-structured situation of the court order. The writer contrasts the position of the probation officer with that of the psychotherapist, 'where', he says, 'voluntary co-operation is assured and where such co-operation is deemed to be indispensable'.[33] The fact, however, that some community hospitals, e.g. JC, have a general catchment area and have a considerable number of patients admitted on a formal basis under sections of the Mental Health Act, would seem to indicate that what he says about the probation service is not totally irrelevant to the psychiatric hospital.

Moffet makes a point similar to that of Studt's: 'Not very long ago "authoritarian" was a word of abuse for case-workers, but opinions have changed and it is now accepted that the case-worker is inevitably an authority figure and must come to terms with the fact.'[34] While not trying to equate the work or position of a social worker with that of hospital staff, nevertheless there are insights that each could usefully share.

If one takes this further and looks at what social workers are doing and saying about the position of the worker in group situations there may well be something of especial value for staffs of a therapeutic community. (See, for example, the article 'Social Worker as Central Person' by K. Heap.)[35] It could be argued that the aims of groups that social workers are likely to be involved in are rather different from the aims of a therapeutic group, and that the approaches are therefore also different. Nevertheless, similarities are apparent as can be seen by comparing the description of the life history of the group and the role of the therapist within it as described by Foulkes and Anthony[36] with a similar threefold pattern that Heap described in his article. And the fact that the former are speaking of group psychotherapy does not necessarily mean that their findings are, in every detail, the more relevant. After all, they are concerned with a very special type of closed, voluntary group. There is room to learn from a wide range of group experience, beyond as well as within the clinical situation.

But to return to the point at which we digressed: that the exercise of authority is possible only where and when others sanction it. This is true where there is a sick situation (the example often quoted is that of Nazi Germany under Hitler) and it is also true in a healthy one, i.e. where there is an exercise of authentic authority. In the one we might say that the relationship is based upon domination and collusion, in the other upon integrity and mutual openness. The problem of how to avoid the one and promote the other is part of the difficulty the therapeutic community tries to tackle, and which it hopes its approaches have a way of solving. Success is never total, for collusion and domination have many and subtle forms, and what appears to be an authentic reciprocity may well be an illusion. But it was in a society of partnership, which may not be a bad way of describing a therapeutic community, that van den Heuvel hoped for a solution to the authority problem, and it is to this that we turn in more detail, looking first at the role of the doctor, then to the question of leadership in the community, especially among the patients.

The one who dares

The title of this section, the one who dares, comes from the writings of Martin Buber in the book *The Knowledge of Man*. He says: 'a "doctor of souls" who really is one – that is, who does not merely carry on the work of healing but enters into it at times as a partner – is precisely one who dares.'[37] In context Buber is speaking specifically to the therapists of the analytical school, telling them of the need to face a situation which may well demand the modification of their methods and the stepping out of the established rules of their school. But it seems quite legitimate to take the idea expressed in this powerful sentence and give it wider application. And initially we will do so in line with Buber's own anthropological thought, speaking as it does not only to the role of doctor in particular but to all in the community set-up.

For Buber 'all real living is meeting', and what makes man distinctively human is his ability to meet other men and his world in a relationship which he has called 'I-Thou'. In his later writings there has been a deepening in his understanding of the ontological basis for his philosophy, and this can be seen in the two-fold movements basic to man which he describes as 'the primal setting at a distance' and 'entering into relation'. The first is the pre-supposition for the second since relationship can only be entered into with that which one has set at a distance allowing it independent existence. And in the relationship of self-with-other experienced in mutual confirmation, co-operation and genuine dialogue the self of each grows. Buber is quite clear that such growth is not achieved in man's relation to himself, in self-realization as 'people like to suppose today', but in relationship with others.

An important word for what makes this relationship real is 'confirmation'. It is used by Buber as being distinctive from two other words often used in therapy and counselling literature namely 'affirmation' and 'acceptance'. This distinction is perhaps made clearest if one compares Buber with Carl Rogers. Put in the most concentrated form, the difference is that whereas Rogers emphasizes 'unqualified acceptance' Buber believes that there must also be a struggle with the other person against himself. This needs unpacking. In the recorded conversation presented at the end of *The Knowledge of Man*, Rogers shows that for him acceptance is of the other person by the man both as he is and as he could be. 'We accept', he says, 'the individual and his potential . . . Acceptance of the most complete sort, acceptance of this person as he is, is the strongest factor making for change that I know. In other words, I think that does release change or release potentiality to find that as I am, I am fully accepted – then I can't help but change.'[38] Buber said he was not so sure of this. He sees in man a polarity which he cannot put aside. 'I have to do with the problematic in him. And there are cases when I must help him against himself. He wants my help against himself.' There is a search for 'redemption' and in trust it is possible for the therapist to help in the struggle involved. And it is this that Buber understands as confirmation as against acceptance. 'I confirm my partner', Buber says, 'as this existing being even while I oppose him.'[39]

Roger's line of thought leads him to think in terms of a full mutuality in the relationship between therapist and client. Buber says that in the helping situation this cannot be so and instead he speaks of 'a one-sided inclusion'. This does not mean that the client is reduced to an object of observation, an It, for the relationship remains one of trust and mutual partnership in a common situation (I-Thou), and indeed this is the only way in which real therapy can take place. But 'a common situation however, does not mean one which each enters from the same or even a similar position'.[40] There is a difference in role and function determined by the very difference of purpose which led each to enter the relationship. 'The full reality of the concrete situation includes the fact that one is a sick man who has come to the therapist for help, the other a therapist who is ready to enter a relationship in order to help.'[41] Speaking to Rogers, Buber says: 'You are able to do something that he is not able. You are not equals and cannot be. You have the great task self-imposed, a great self-imposed task to supplement this need of his and do rather more than in the normal situation. But, of course, there are limits, and I may be allowed to tell you certainly in your experience as a therapist, as a healing person or helping to healing you must experience it again and again, the limits to simple humanity.'[42]

Confirming is not, for Buber, merely a therapeutic technique: it is involved in all real dialogue and all authentic meeting. One of the factors that makes for inauthentic meeting is what he describes as 'seeming' as against 'being'. The 'seeming' man proceeds in his relationships with others from a calculation of what will meet approval, from a concern with how he will 'seem' to others, what his image is. The 'being' man, however, is concerned with no such calculation but just gives himself without thought of the image presented. It is recognized that these are generally found in mixture. To yield to seeming is man's essential cowardice and to resist it is his essential courage, in a struggle that is never in vain.

My own feeling is that Buber's approach, sketchily and inadequately outlined here, affords a valuable source for dialogue across several disciplines – philosophy, theology and psychiatry for example. But these are wider issues and for the immediate purpose I want to look at just four points: relationship for wholeness, the struggle 'against', the inequalities of the common situation, and the 'being' man.

It would not be possible here to enter into the debate concerning just what it is that either 'causes' or proves therapeutic in cases of mental illness. It is sufficient to say that in the therapeutic communities there is seldom a complete rejection of the physical aspects but that the importance of the influence of relationships underlies much of the therapeutic attitudes. The aim is that both staff and patients meet in the mutual and open relationship of person to person, and this involves risk, for to be open with another is to lay oneself open to the risk of change and rejection. This means that it is not only the doctor but everyone in the place are people that must 'dare'. But the traditional structuring of relationships between patient and doctor have kept fairly firm defences around the doctor such that he is kept as far as possible from existential risk. The patient is 'set at a distance' and kept there in a position of the one who is observed, in an I-It relation. The doctor is the one who examines the patient, records a mental and physical 'history', diagnoses, prescribes, is detached. All these are necessary, but this can harden into a fixed polarity which severely limits the open mutuality of the real shared situation. Out of this, there cannot be real meeting, nor, I would suggest, that level of healing which looks towards 'wholeness'.

The open mutuality that is sought for in the doctor/patient relationship is not merely a mutuality that takes and leaves the other as he is. There is acceptance in the sense that the patient is accepted as this person with this individual existence towards whom one does not adopt a moralistic, crushing attitude. On the community level such acceptance finds expression in the use of the word permissive. As with so many other ideological words, this is by no means as precise a notion as might be thought. Even the community that makes use of the word is also conscious of limits to its application, yet without being sure in the concrete situation just what criteria are used to set those limits. Take, for example, destructive or disturbed behaviour. Individual acts may be permitted (i.e. allowed to go unsanctioned, though at best not unconfronted), yet at some point a limit is felt to be crossed and action becomes necessary. The final incident that prompts action (denial of outdoor clothes, putting to bed, etc.) may in itself be no different from any one of the previous incidents that went by relatively unheeded, but the limit is reached when the community members – doctors, nurses or patients, or all together, feel that it can stand no more, either for its own good or, and one suspects that this is quite often second, for the patient's good. There are limits, therefore, to the non-judgmental and the permissive code, both with the individual and the community. And it is right as well as common-sense that it should be so. A. Storr has pointed this out in the context of the family and the school: 'In a regime in which rebellion is impossible since everything is tolerated, there is less scope for the individual to develop than one in which the teachers as well as the pupils have their rights.'[43]

In his relationship with the patient, therefore, the doctor is not only emphatically conscious of these elements in the other which are self-negating, destructive, unreal, etc., but is with the patient in the struggle against them. It may well be part of his role to help the patient to become aware of them as destructive, etc., and to support the fight against them. The danger in this, of course, is that the doctor forsakes the dialogical 'struggle with' and retires to the monologue of a dominating word of judgment backed up by the formal authority of his place in the social structure.

This latter problem is all the more severe if one accepts the Buber idea that although the relationship between the doctor and patient is one of open mutuality, there remains by the very necessity of the concrete situation a one-sidedness about it. Buber is very careful to explain just what he means by this, distinguishing between the fact of the concrete situation and subjective feeling in the therapist. Care is certainly needed for otherwise what one attempts to escape from, in struggling free of the rigid defences of formal authority, catches up on one in more subtle guises. But what it seems to me Buber is saying is that there are formal elements in the situation which cannot be denied and which it is an illusion to deny. While these may not be the over-riding or determining factors in the relationship they nevertheless remain and play some part.

Some therapists, especially of the psychoanalytical school, have given a special stress to the element of authority in the one-sidedness and seen here the main element of the therapeutic process. In *Counselling and Psychotherapy: Theory and Practice*, C. H. Patterson has a section on authority in which he has this to say: 'Authority has been seen by many as a common element, even as the major element in psychotherapy. The therapist is and must be, it is argued, an authority figure.' Tracing the development of psychoanalysis from hypnosis, which he describes as 'authoritative in nature,' Patterson goes on to state how this was replaced by suggestion and other authoritative methods such as reassurance, persuasion, advice, manipulation, etc., and he gives quotes from De Grazia, whom he describes as 'perhaps the most explicit advocates of authority as the essential element in psychotherapy'.[44] 'The following circumstances which establish the authoritative nature of the relationship', says Dr Grazia, 'are to be found in all known psychotherapies. First of all, the patient is in grave need, the therapist is not . . . the patient is ignorant, whereas the therapist is informed . . . the patient expects to be obedient as passive while the therapist is to be active, to tell him what to do . . . Furthermore the patient believes that disobedience to the therapist carries a penalty. Translated into concrete terms the prestige of the therapist insures that in matters of dress, achievement, language, income, education, taste or manners, the patient generally will feel that he is dealing with someone of higher status.'[45] It may well be felt that his is going too far and reveals the very dangers group therapists see in one-to-one therapy, but there are elements here that cannot be ignored, and those who work in therapeutic communities might do well to examine how far they play an unrecognized part in the relationships between staff and patients.

The given factors of the situation and roles of the doctor/patient relationship provide ample opportunity for both doctor and patient to retreat into the 'cowardly' defence of 'seeming'. The doctor works from the exalted position of his formal status and remains 'over' the patient who is 'under' him. The one plays out his role of superiority and the other of submissive dependency. They relate in terms of what is expected of such roles and generalize their role of expectations. Thus the doctor is sought out as an authority, not merely on medical matters but on almost anything. As a doctor said in a recent TV programme, people come to us on almost all problems, much as they used to go to the priest. The relationship between the two authorities is very interesting and, at a time when the cult of health has for many replaced the religion of salvation, it is not surprising that for those who seek the prepared answer, the authoritative reply, for the doctor who is rushed, who dare not risk losing the faith of his followers, who is grateful for the strength afforded by his status so that no one will guess where his weakness lies, there is every temptation to fulfil the expected role. Submissive dependence gets what it asks for – domination. But the doctor who 'dares' moves beyond those aspects of his role which endorse his 'seeming', his public image, and although he may not escape them completely, seeks to meet his patient as this person here and now, as one who dares to 'be'.

We have tended to speak so far in this section as though the doctor/patient relationship were a one-to-one affair. For many in the medical service this is of course the case. But a noted feature of the community is that apart from an initial interview and others occasionally here and there, the doctor/patient relationship is always in the context of the group. How far then does this invalidate what has been said? As far as the material from Buber is concerned it is true that in the past he has had little to say about group relationships and, indeed, at one time denied that his ideas on dialogue and meeting could be applied to the group situation. Latterly, however, he has changed this position somewhat and not only believes that groups can be the places of real meeting but has also developed ideas of wider mutual relationships which could be pertinent – see especially his ideas in the chapter on 'What is common to all'.[46] And in so far as in the therapeutic community 'all' are 'therapists', much of what he says is very relevant, although in practice far from easy to act upon.

The special problem for the doctor in the community is that the nature of his authority is played out along many different lines, and in avoiding the inappropriate use of his authority both in terms of his formal position and as a person (e.g. as just a member of the group) he, more than almost any other, is seeking to remain on the knife edge between authoritarianism and abdication. Formally his authority rests in the obvious facts such as his medical knowledge, his position in the hierarchy, his legal responsibility with regard to section patients, drugs, etc. Informally there is the whole range of role expectation which comes from patients and the rest of the staff. Within the groups the doctor seeks to be just another member of the group – one of the people there. In the large groups this is probably very difficult but may be possible in the smaller groups. Instead of being DOCTOR or DOCTOR Smith, he can come to be seen as Dr Smith or even Dr JOHN SMITH, though it is idle to think he will ever be JOHN SMITH.

Every incentive is given to the group to come to its own decisions rather than to rely on the 'word' of the doctor. There is in fact a positive policy of refusing to provide 'authoritative' answers to strings of patients' questions. The rationale for this is to be found in part in the belief that the problem of authority is one common to most of the patients, related of course to past experience with parents, etc., but also in the belief that the decision which really means something is the decision in which the persons involved have an active part to play. Further, the making of decisions requires a level of information about the relevant facts. The common belief seems to be that a medical man (or any authority figure for that matter) can make right decisions off the top of his head, or perhaps rather that by virtue of his position, past education, etc., he has a degree of omniscience which means he comes to decisions without the normal means of information gathering. This is clearly unreal, and doctors rightly refuse (or they are right when they refuse) to collude with this by a declaration which is aimed at confirming the illusion entertained. The alternative is either to sit in silent refusal to answer at all or to refer the matter to the group. The latter is preferable, and especially so when the information sought is available from the group resources. This not only affirms the democratic nature of decision making but at best arrives at a more rounded picture of the situation and therefore a more real decision.

An example of this would be the common one of a patient asking the doctor if he can have his clothes back. The appeal to the doctor is based on the assumption that (*a*) he was the one to order the patient to have his clothes taken from him (i.e. acted as judge, since this is often seen as a punishment), (*b*) he alone has the authority to rescind the order, (*c*) he is in the best position, (i.e. he is the best informed to make the decision), (*d*) that whatever anyone else will say the doctor's decision is final anyway. The complexity of even this simple situation arises in part because there is a mixture of fact and illusion in the assumption.

(*a*) If the clothes were taken off the patient on admission, rather than later, when it is more likely to have been a group decision, then the chances are that the situation demanded that the doctor make an immediate decision and it was in fact on his authority that the clothes were removed. There is a clear distinction, of course, between the removal of clothes from someone to prevent his leaving the unit and their removal for cleaning, but this is not always clear to the patient. The patient thus seeks remission from the person who 'condemned', or if the decision was taken lower down the hierarchy at a time of crisis, then addressing the doctor is an appeal to higher court.

(*b*) This follows by assumption but not in fact. Quite a large number of decisions have to be made by an authoritative person without recourse to a group, but where there is room for a change that decision can be questioned and revoked by a group. This is not realized because there is a fallacy in the thinking of point (*c*).

(*c*) While the doctor may well know more of the background and clinical history of the patient, he is less likely to know more than the other patients about the general behaviour and relationships the patient has built up, and therefore it is they who are in a better position to pool information as to whether or not the patient would be likely to run off or be destructive were he to have his clothes back.

(*d*) Ideally this too is fallacious, and yet there will almost inevitably be circumstances when it is necessary for a doctor to have to assert his formal authority. At best these should be explained as particular circumstances rather than left as the basis for generalization, but it is not always easy to do. There is thus, in all this, some ambiguity.

And the doctors are very conscious of the ambiguity of their own situation, part of which is implicit in what was said much earlier with regard to the differential diffusion of authority and responsibility. For therapeutic reasons it may be important that a group of patients be given or afforded the authority to decide any number of matters concerning the running of the community, and the doctor is pleased to delegate this authority. But the responsibility in certain spheres remains with him and his colleagues, and this is the source of potential tension and conflict, in both the community and himself. This in itself is not necessarily a bad thing if it is made the basis for a learning situation. It can become destructive if left by default or made the basis for a sudden reversal to authoritarian decisions.

As a member of a group the doctor is consciously playing down his authority position in its formal sense. It is possible, however, for this to reach exaggerated proportions. While on any number of topics he is clearly no more a necessary authority than others who are present, yet there remain areas of knowledge and opinion where by training and experience he is an authority. Clearly on matters of factual medical information this is so. An *a priori* refusal to answer straight questions in this sphere seems to me clearly unrealistic. Yet it must be admitted that there is a caution to be exercised in allowing a group to stall from its real work by the setting up of various medical questions to be answered by the doctor expert.

The therapeutic purpose requires a parsimonious care of the ready answer, but it might be questionable (other staff certainly do question it) when the same thing appears in the face of nursing questions, for example. The generalization is both exaggerated and unfair, but I have heard nurses often say that 'in this place you can never get anyone to make a decision or give a straight answer'. While the medical staff are often the focus of this complaint it also has general application and seems to be felt by some to be the price that has to be paid for working in the community set-up. At times, of course, the doctor is put in an unreal position by the staff in much the same way as he is by the patients.

This is especially true of the consultants. Staff continue to appeal to consultant authority on a range of topics that are well outside the strictly medical areas and which the consultant is not necesarily the one who is or can be the authority. There is a similarity between the patient who places himself under the doctor and demands decisions from him yet refuses to carry all of them out (e.g. demands drugs yet refuses the medication provided) and the staff who appeal to the consultants for a decision yet meet the decision with complaints on the grounds that it was not a group decision. Such a situation can become very complex and would appear to be associated with times of most severe pressure and anxiety. Stanton and Schwarz note as a general fact that where the 'culture' of the hospital is 'anti-formal' the attitude to the formal tends to be one of rebellion against a call for formality to meet certain problems.[47] There is something of wanting the cake and eating it and, in a community that emphasizes the informal approaches yet by necessity still has aspects of the formal within it, this tendency seems to be a fairly marked form of defence system.

But not all the appeals for leadership from the consultant are unreal. The staff do not merely ask for ready-made decisions from the big boss but something more complex and less easy to define. There is the search for leadership in which to have confidence, a sense of purposeful movement. And when all due qualifications have been made, there is a desire for some sort of consistency between the informal ideology and the actual actions and decisions made. Harsh as it may be, one nevertheless hears a complaint of 'two-facedness' – the seen contradiction between broad informal statements of intent and the particular acts made in the face of crisis or formal responsibility. Consultants do not any more than others have a magic formula with which to solve the problems created by the tension between formal responsibilities and informal ideologies, but because they are in a position of particular vulnerability it is probably incumbent upon them to be more than usually vigilant. Those nearest to the consultant, i.e. registrars and senior registrars, are most likely to be affected by any inconsistency here and also most likely to be critical.

One hesitates at suggesting even the most general line that might assist in the easing of the 'doctor's dilemma' in this area. For if the findings of Rapaport at the Belmont Unit have any wider validity, it would seem that authority and responsibility are focal points for a doctor in coming to terms with the role he has to play in the therapeutic community. 'If any single set of dilemmas can be designated as focal in stimulating the emergent patterns of performance in doctors' roles, it is probably the set arising from the area of authority–responsibility. In the doctor's role more than in any of the others, there is a marked discrepancy between the formal basis for authority and expectations with regard to responsibility on the one hand and the Unit's ideological tenets on the other. This discrepancy makes itself felt and must be dealt with in all the doctor's activities. His pattern of role performance hinges to a very great extent on how he resolves the dilemmas implied in this discrepancy.[48]

It would seem to me important that in an 'informal' society and culture due weight should be given to the place and influence of those aspects of the formal that remain to play their part. The danger seems to be much less that informality will be whittled away by the edge of rigid restructuring, than that the formal aspects that persist both below and above the surface should be implicitly ignored. Failure to take them into real account may well be a source of frustration and tension centred upon the doctor. What we have called 'abdication' is less likely to be the basis of criticism than the retreat into authoritarianism, and to that extent it needs even more careful watching.

But appropriate decision making, the taking of responsibility, speaking 'as one with authority' do not necessarily mean an authoritarian attitude even though position and status and not merely this man as this man, is involved.

We have called the doctor the man who dares. Among the traditional such a call to open authentic person-to-person meeting in an I-Thou relationship no doubt seems to be either an idle dream of those with too much time to spare or a threat to the dignity of a professional status. To the 'existentialist' it is the radical trumpet call to a freedom beyond all that is formal and structured to that involvement where persons interact out of the given moment with spontaneity and ever fresh insight. But to the doctor of the therapeutic community it is a call which searches for the openness of real meeting amidst the recognition of expectations, pre-conceived and learnt role images, and amidst the reality of the 'one-sided inclusion'. For this is a part of the given situation in which he seeks to play an authentic, health-helping, illuminating role.

Leadership among 'equals'

The discussion of the role of the doctor and previously that concerning the staff hierarchy has attempted to show that an ideology of 'equality' does not necessarily exclude an authentic form of authority and responsibility exercised upon both formal and informal levels. One is conscious that it may appear that the slogan 'All men are equal' is being underwritten again by 'but some are more equal than others'. It is right that this barb should bite if a society lives by a practice that belies its preaching. Nevertheless it may be a little more than a superficial jibe if the complexity of the word 'equal' is not appreciated. Equality as a rallying cry is common both in the employment and the political arenas, but the meaning of the word has to be found in its contextual setting and its evocative value seems all too often to be proportional to the vagueness of its use. Equal what? we must ask. Equal physique? equal ability? equal rights? equal value? To call, for example, for 'equal education for all' could in fact result in an education policy that makes nonsense of the intentions of the reformers. So too the appeal to the equality of man may be no more than a cover for the reduction of men to a numerical collective. And it may equally be the basis for an extreme individualism which leads to a dreadful isolation. In philosophical anthropology, theology and psychology we can find examples of the pendulum swinging to these extremes. The struggle to find a realistic via media is no easy matter. Buber's individualism of 'I-Thou' was necessarily modified by the exploration of the 'essential WE'. Protestant individualism has been set in a truer perspective by a renewed emphasis upon the setting within the community. The isolated client of psychoanalysis is seen to be better understood and better helped to wholeness in a familial or group context.

If we then speak of 'equals' in a therapeutic community we must do so with due regard to the context and the qualifications the word needs from its general vague use. It clearly does not mean a formal equality but rather something like the equality of rights to voice an opinion and to be given a significant hearing. In a culture that gives special emphasis to verbal communication this seems one possible way of understanding the word. In connection with leadership this finds expression in the freedom within the groups and community for authority to rest with those who are not formally seen as in any particular position of the status structure. Leadership then becomes not a matter of the pre set patterns but of the way in which people relate in open, common situations. In the group meeting there is no predetermining of who will in fact be the leader at any given moment, authority resting with him who speaks with authority, be it patient, domestic cleaner, doctor, social worker or visitor.

In so far as he or she has 'some apparent controlling power' to which the rest 'submit' in reciprocal sanctioning, he is for that time the one with authority, the leader. And it is from this interchange of relationships that the group that is unstructured finds a structure. For it to remain authentic and not dominating there must be openness and fluidity about this pattern, and so it is that the leadership role moves from one to another.

The retreat of authority-persons from the open creative use of a leadership role in the face of anxiety is, of course, a special tempta-tion for the staff, since they have a safely prepared hideyhole within the formal structure should the need arise. But something similar can also be seen among patients. Even when authority is not for-malized in such roles as community or ward chairman, implicit structures can appear beneath the surface built on such factors as length of stay, experience of ECT (so often referred to as The Treat-ment), membership of a particular doctor's team, admission at other hospitals in the past, as well as the wider social factors like age, sex, marriage, education and so on. A quite common pheno-menon especially among the more experienced and intelligent is the adoption of a pseudo-staff role which attempts to bring to the authority of the individual the overshadowing of a wider and 'higher' authority. At one level this may appear in the habit of repeating to the group in general the remark just made by a member of staff. A little more subtly the remark is not merely repeated but reworded and partially interpreted. The adoption of psychological terminology goes along with this. Such leadership may resort to a technique of a type of round robin enquiry after everybody's health or the more powerful method, because less stereotyped and showing more concern, of being father-confessor or mother-comforter to the group.

It would be wrong to suggest that all such incidents of leadership are destructive or unhealthy. The group can and sometimes does use them to work with, and patients do often make valuable contri-butions in the process of 'role-acting'. But in practice, because they usually indicate a retreat of this person from facing his own prob-lems into a role of dominating the course of the group's proceedings away from his own anxiety areas, such occasions often result in a shift of leadership to a person who interprets what is going on so that the deposed leader may learn from the event. Sometimes it is patients that fill this role, but it is more often staff, especially in larger groups, who fulfil this role of interpreter, if it is felt that the group as a whole is colluding in an inauthentic leadership.

Community anxiety can be seen not only in the exercise of authority but in the appeal to authority as well. In a place like the Conolly, where there are no real facilities for the enforced control of disturbed or violent patients, outbreaks of violence arouse special anxieties among patients and staff. From the patients' point of view the matter is for staff authority to do something about, and the anxiety sometimes expresses itself in strong anti-staff attitudes and complaints that the staff are failing in their duty. It is not uncommon to find that the patient body finds a spokesman to express its feelings, formally in the role of the chairman or informally through someone who is commonly vocal in staff criticism. The responsibility of a sort of mutual care that the patients have for one another and which is encouraged by the staff is felt to be overburdened and the sanctions of punishment controlled by the staff are sought for – removal of clothes, confining to bed, increased medication, transferral, etc. Staff reaction to such requests would seem to be founded on a number of considerations. Patient anxiety may be unreal in face of the actual overt acts committed and there is then the need for the situation to be examined and the relationships involved brought to light for therapeutic purposes. The level of staff anxiety is also a factor – it would appear that violence to property is less anxiety-provoking than violence to the patient himself (suicide attempts, for example, always carry fairly high anxiety levels), but if the property is large enough (large electrical equipment, for example), action is also likely. Among domestic and catering staff more minor breakages probably are sufficient to raise anxieties, since the areas of responsibility are more closely attached to matters of equipment. Persistent and destructive group blocking is also likely to lead to authoritative action. Destructiveness that puts a long-term strain on nursing staff is liable to be given as a reason for transferral attempts with a rationale found in the unsuitability of the hospital architecture. In all this, both with patients and staff, there is a mixture of the real and the unreal and it is probably not possible to find clear-cut criteria for the resultant decisions. The association of such incidents with a crisis-like situation means that at such times there is perhaps a more than usual willingness to allow and expect decisions to be made from those of senior status.

Reference was made earlier to formal patient responsibility in the shape of community and ward chairmen. Until recently, at the JC these posts were part of the community structure. Their disappearance in the last few months is evidence that there is some question about their value. The debate in fact continues at least under the surface and behind the scenes since some of the staff feel that such positions were of benefit to patients and the community. In part at least it would seem to be a question of the reality of a staff-imposed system of responsibility on the one hand and the value of a formal focus of leadership on the other. Those who favour their disappearance would argue that the chairman structure was in fact imposed upon the patients rather than evolved from the situation and from the feelings of the patients themselves, and that it was therefore in some ways an alien form of leadership. It also meant that at community meetings, for example, some degree of structure was pre-arranged for the meeting, especially when it was linked with a formal system of feeding-in information. In some units, the place of the community meeting would appear to be almost sacrosanct as an essential part of what it means to be a therapeutic community. For various reasons this has been questioned at the JC, though it remains a tense debating point. It is yet to be seen whether the gains are found to outweigh the disadvantages of not having daily meetings of the whole community. It is possible that what was hoped for was a patient-evolved pattern of responsibility, informal and therefore more real, or formalized in ways decided upon by the patients themselves. It is true that some of the patients are willing to take on responsibility – e.g. to help new patients to settle in, showing visitors around, helping with the sick, etc., but in a quick turn-over population it might be questioned how far any pattern actually develops.

Part of the value of the formal system was the fact that responsibility by the patients within the community was an openly discussed matter. The election of either ward or community chairman may well have appeared on the surface as something of a farce. The call for nominations all too often resulted in a whole list of proposed candidates promptly followed by a succession of refusals to accept nomination. Actual voting for the candidates who did accept often relied less on assessment by patients of the candidate than on the call to vote. Thus, on several occasions at the JC, it happened that not only did people vote for two opposing candidates but switched their vote when a re-vote was called for. It might be concluded from this that there was no real sense of responsibility in the community or that there was a sort of acting out of the reaction to an imposed system. Nevertheless, it could also be argued that it was of value to be able to confront patients with their desire to avoid a position of responsibility and also provided for those who were elected a valuable learning situation.

I have heard it said, for example, that a team felt it would be helpful to a particular patient if he were to take on the role of chairman. It is true that there is a danger that the formalization of yet another 'authority' figure provides a further crutch for those patients to lean upon when they are unwilling to stand on their own two feet. But it is probably also true that chairmen encouraged greater degrees of responsibility among the other patients in matters that directly concerned the management of wards, the care of visitors, etc. Without ward chairmen, for example, the role of encouraging patients to keep ward areas and kitchens tidy falls on the staff, and it is more likely to be seen as a staff requirement rather than something for which the ward itself was responsible. And this leads to the tendency to rely on those patients who are willing horses rather than to confront all patients with areas of responsibility.

At its widest level this problem focuses a difficulty about the limits to be put on the idea of the 'unstructured'. Just as in the question of the hierarchy and of the authority of the doctor, it seems necessary to give due recognition to those elements which are to some extent anti the general culture of the place, i.e. the place of the hierarchy even when it is flattened and the formal aspects of authority amidst the authentic informal aspects, so too I think that it should be recognized that there are considerable areas of a patient's life which are laid down for him and that this is not only necessary but has a positive value which, though open to abuse, can also be used. Those who support the chairman system as at least one form of patient responsibility might well argue that it is just such a one of the valuable structures.

CONCLUSIONS

It is in some senses invidious to attempt to draw out conclusions from something which I have felt all along has been more in the way of exploration of my own understanding and experience of a therapeutic community than the setting out of evidence for certain hypotheses. Nevertheless, I have been conscious of one or two general lines of thought. The first is that for all the difficulties and for all the criticisms in detail that may have been made, I realize that my bias is very much in favour of the therapeutic community. It is a bias rather than part of a creed because my experience of psychiatric hospitals is one-sided. But I end up very much with the feeling that here is a way of authentic meeting and caring which attempts to see men whole. It has not solved all the problems thrown up by the traditional methods; indeed it has thrown up many of its own, yet it holds a potential for real learning, real communication and real healing, in a way which I can only describe as more truly human.

The second point is this: that in seeking to overcome the dangers and faults of the past approaches which seem now at odds with the community ideology and culture, there are manifold problems in finding criteria for describing the limits of such aspects of the ideology as permissiveness, democracy, informal responsibility and authority, and the 'unstructured' situation. With this goes the need that those elements of sanction, autocracy, formality and structure that remain should be openly recognized and used to positive benefit rather than apologized for or kept by tension under the surface. Recognition of the extent, dangers and values of both sets of factors is necessary for an appreciation of the complexity of the situation and the way it actually is. If allowed to go unrecognized the possible tensions between the two will gnaw with aggravation at each other under the surface to appear in fantastic form at times of any increase in anxiety.

And the third point is simply that since it would seem to me that one of the great values of the therapeutic community is its willingness to risk the anxiety of probing forward in the search for better approaches and greater knowledge, without the false security of believing that the truth has been found, the temptation of establishing a settled approach or conforming to any one model needs to be continually faced. So too does the temptation at times of change to look to a golden past that in fact never existed – whether it be the past of traditionalism or the past of a community pattern now superseded. Lot's wife should be a warning to all who indulge in this pastime!

If it has seemed that I have continually wandered from the topic of authority as such, I have to admit that it is so. And yet it has seemed to me that the problem of authority is what lies behind so many of the difficulties and possibilities of the therapeutic communities. Together with anxiety, it forms one of the characteristics not only of the hospital but of any social organism, and their relationship and interaction inevitably spider-web their way through an intricate, involved and fascinating network.

NOTES

1. See e.g. Freud, *On the Nature of Jokes and their Relation to the Unconscious*

2. R. W. Revans, *Standards for Morale*, OUP 1964, p. 91

3. D. Cooper, 'The Anti-hospital', *New Society*, 11 March 1965

4. On the treatment of schizophrenics see J. Willis, *Lecture-notes on Psychiatry*, Blackwell 1968, Ch. 3

5. D. Martin, *A Sociology of English Religion*, Heinemann and SCM Press 1967, p. 65

6. H. H. Perlman, 'The Role Concept and Social Casework', *New Developments in Casework*, ed. E. Younghusband, Allen and Unwin 1966, p. 64

7. W. J. Goode, *The Family*, Prentice-Hall 1964, p. 4

8. Elements in this process such as an over-domineering father, passive mother, or the reverse, will be likely to have adverse consequences in an individual's later relations to authority figures

9. R. W. Revans, op. cit., see thesis as outlined in introduction

10. See e.g. R. N. Rapaport, *Community as Doctor*, Tavistock Publications 1960, Appendix A, p. 306

11. I. Menzies, 'A Case-study in the functioning of Social Systems as a Defence Against Anxiety', *Human Relations*, Vol. 13, 1960

12. N. Exchaquet, 'Role of the Head Nurse in the Management of the Ward', *International Nursing Review*, Sept./Oct. 1967

13. I. Menzies, op. cit., p. 105

14. Theological parallels can be found for this

15. A. Stanton and M. Schwarz, *The Mental Hospital*, Basic Books 1954

16. R. W. Revans, op. cit., p. xii

17. R. W. Revans, op. cit., p. 91

18. R. W. Revans, op. cit., p. x

19. M. Jones, *Social Psychiatry*, Tavistock Publications 1952

20. R. W. Revans, op. cit., p. 92

21. A. Camus, *The Plague*, Penguin 1960, p. 182

22. R. N. Rapaport, op. cit., p. 73

23. R. W. Revans, op. cit., p. xv

24. A. H. van den Heuvel, *The Humiliation of The Church*, SCM Press 1967, p. 153

25. D. H. Clark, *Administrative Therapy*, Tavistock Publications 1964, p. 109

26. See D. Knowles, *Evolution of Medieval Thought*, Longmans 1962

27. D. Cooper, op. cit.

28. Dr J. C. N. Tibbits, 'Notes for a Paper on the Concept of Authority' (unpublished)

29. D. Cooper, op. cit.

30. E. Studt, 'Worker-client Authority Relationships in Social Work' in Younghusband, p. 176 (see 6 above)

31. J. Moffet, *Concepts in Casework Treatment*, Routledge & Kegan Paul 1968, p. 77

32. E. Studt, op. cit. (see 6 above)

33. A. Hunt, 'Enforcement in Probation Casework,' in Younghusband, pp. 156-7 (see 6 above)

34. J. Moffet, op. cit., p. 70

35. K. Heap, 'Social Worker as Central Person', in *Social Work*, Jan. 1968

36. Foulkes and Anthony, *Group Psychotherapy*, Penguin 1957

37. M. Buber, *The Knowledge of Man*, Allen and Unwin 1965, p. 123

38. M. Buber, op. cit., p. 182

39. M. Buber, op. cit., p. 183
40. M. Buber, op. cit., Introductory essay by M. Friedman, p. 31
41. M. Buber, op. cit., Introductory essay by M. Friedman, p. 32
42. M. Buber, op. cit., p. 172
43. A. Storr, *The Integrity of the Personality*, Penguin 1963, p. 94
44. C. H. Patterson, *Counseling and Psychotherapy: Theory and Practice*, Harper & Row 1959, pp. 297 ff.
45. De Grazia, *Errors of Psychotherapy*, Doubleday & Co., New York 1952, p. 103
46. M. Buber, op. cit., Ch. 4
47. Stanton and Schwarz, op. cit.
48. Rapaport, op. cit., p. 118

6 Difficult Patients and Difficult Doctors

1   R. E. D. Markillie
2   A. R. Anderson

This chapter is composed of two addresses delivered at the 1968 Assembly of the Institute of Religion and Medicine at Oxford. The general title was 'Communication and Health'.

The first part is by Dr R. E. D. Markillie, a Consultant Psychiatrist and Lecturer in Psychiatry at Leeds University.

The second part is by Dr A. R. Anderson, who is not a medical doctor but a physical chemist at the Atomic Energy Research Establishment at Harwell.

1

As this section, 'Difficult Patients and Difficult Doctors', is part of the whole concept of communication and health, let us assume that we are talking about communication in or about bad health or threatened health, or something that purports to be either of these. Let us also assume that we are in a supply and demand equation. As there are hens and eggs, there have always been patients and doctors however they may have been named. Hence no communication ever occurs about health, or bad health in particular, without expectations certainly on the part of the needy, and more than one might expect on the part of the helpers too. Those expectations play a very great part in difficulties on either side. For example, medical or psychiatric jokes, and the musical hall question 'Is there a doctor in the house?' with its consequences, all imply the existence of expectations.

That leads me to a proposition. *Only when the expectations of the one party more or less match what the other party has to offer is the transaction stress-free and possibly results in relief and cure.* There I am not specifying which are helpers and doctors, for the transaction works both ways. Quite clearly in medicine much communication arouses no problems whatever. One example that I regularly use in teaching is the situation in which someone walks in with a whitlow. He holds up a finger about twice the size of a normal one, a horrible purple-grey colour, and nobody really needs to say anything, or ask any questions. The need is apparent at once. Or if someone is brought in off the road, having been smashed up, then again there are no problems about communication, or relatively few. And from the accounts that many of us have heard from our missionary friends of the work that they do with an enormous quantity of untreated and very gross disease which produces great suffering – again there are few communication problems.

The thing begins to become a problem in our changing culture with our changing cultural values. If I suggest that there is a progressive alienation from the personal, that is a hypothesis, and no clear evaluation has been done on it. But illness has, so to speak, been sucked into man's personal dis-ease, and different types of message now get communicated within it, and about it, very different from the ones that I have just mentioned.

Now let us look at this in quite another way for a minute. If you were to prepare a histogram in which your ordinates were all the types of difficulty between patients and doctors and the frequency of their occurrence, I am sure you would find the peak of that curve (in other words what most frequently occurs) to be a wide band containing a group of patient–doctor encounters in which there was a failure of communication in the sense that what was being offered by the patient was not acceptable to the doctor, or not understood by him in the terms in which the offer was made, or vice versa. Another type of failure would be that the doctor was operating in terms of a model of treatment of a patient when there was really no patient, or that the presumed patient was not seeking treatment but seeking something else. Another, and quite different, situation might arise when the doctor appears to be occupying a healing role, but when in fact he is not. I shall try to amplify some of these in a few minutes.

Let me switch to a non-clinical example to make my point clearer – to a clerical example, and here I must try to keep myself tightly to role and not introduce my own ideas on this example. If you consider confession and absolution I think you will see an example of what I mean when I say that you cannot absolve a morbid delusion of guilt. It may look like one thing but it is not what it seems to be;

and this is one of the things which certainly creates difficulties for the clergy, and comparable examples create difficulty for the doctor. I have used the word 'offered' but I think 'proffered' is etymologically more exact. Now there is nothing new or progressive in talking about offers. Michael Balint wrote about this delightfully clearly in 1957,[1] but it is a lesson that I find I am being reminded daily still needs to be learned. Again and again it comes up in one's experience with doctors and in talking with them about patients that they have problems in treating. Some of the doctors in the first seminar that Michael Balint ran at the Tavistock Clinic framed the following questions about the basic difficulties in handling their patients.

1. *What does the patient need from the doctor and what does he actually get?* This is a question seldom enough asked, though maybe many of our patients in fact have got jolly good answers to it if only you ask them the question. Should not the clergy ask it of themselves and of their clients?

2. *What is it that the doctor gives the patient that the patient does not want or need?* One short partial answer to that is several millions pounds worth of unused drugs; quite apart from the useless ones, of which there are several millions pounds worth more. Again the clergy should ask themselves the same question.

Let me exemplify what I have said by listing a few types of difficult patient and difficult doctor, but talking of it again from the point of principle rather than biographical accounts. Difficult patients first. *The patient who proffers illness to gain some social sanction and therefore fails to respond as expected to the treatment persistently applied.* To use a value judgment I could split those into good and bad. The good profferings of illness to gain social sanction, the understandable ones; and the ones that we would call skiving or miking or swinging the lead.

You might call a good one the miner who works in impossible and frightening conditions. He becomes afraid and can only cope with this fear by becoming ill. I think one might say this about the skiving although perhaps it is a little unfair. Just watch the newspapers; when anybody wealthy is wanted for fraud he is nearly always ill with a heart attack or his doctors have sent certificates saying that he cannot travel for three months, or something of the sort. If you keep tabs on this kind of thing, you will see illness being used to gain a social sanction and perhaps an advantage.

Another type of difficult patient is *the one who wants his spice and his halfpenny.* This is a human enough wish but one which medical skill cannot satisfy. Such patients may anger their doctors if they keep on asking for this or if afterwards they do not pay because they did not get the unreal expectation.

Very close to that last one is *the patient looking for magic, an omnipotent and totally unreal Nobodaddy; the patient who cannot face the unknown, the uncertainty, who wants an answer, a diagnosis –* '*What does the book say?*' Now there are many of those. If the patient has got a whitlow it is very easy to say what is wrong with him, but when his life is all haywire how can you? Such patients are very common indeed and become more common in times of national or world uncertainty. And when such a one meets a doctor who cannot face just those same things himself (and many of them obviously cannot any more than their patients can) then there is likely to be trouble. Both are going to be accusing each other of being difficult doctors or difficult patients as the case may be and complaining to their friends and colleagues.

Now if it may seem that I am lambasting doctors in this, let me redress the balance a little and say something that may be controversial but which I very deeply believe myself. Doctors fall for such demands with monotonous regularity because it flatters us to be regarded as omnipotent. But, I think, so do some clergy.

I cannot help thinking that some of those who concretize the sacraments and offer them as sovereign remedies for the discomforts, even the persecution and the uncertainties in life, or to reduce the enormous gap between our view and our experience of life and God's purpose which belongs to the life of faith, do just the same. I cannot help feeling that there is something of the same kind of omnipotence being sought and offered in that aside from the human concern of God or the theological basis of the ministry. There is this plea to us again and again to do something which in fact we cannot do. We, doctors and clergy, respond to the dependent plea from the patient to do something while he, the patient, does nothing. He tries to hand a baby smartly to you. Some babies you can take, but the babies that usually get handed to you are the ones that nobody else wants either. This leads to the so-called difficult patient. One of the curses of traditional medical education is that doctors are trained to be doers not teachers, not working with the docile, not drawers out or leaders out of things from their patients, but doers, and patients often seduce us into being doers where angels would fear to tread.

Now for some difficult doctors. This list may seem at first to be value judgments but it is easier to put it pithily. *The selfish* – those who are in it for gold, or perhaps in it for status, the lazy or the slothful who think it is easier to deal with things than people. Obviously it is, but it is people whom we are called upon to deal with. *The sick* (and there are many kinds of sick doctors) – the opinionated; the omnipotent; the Messianic.

Let me quote a piece from a somewhat unlikely source about a failure of communication between doctor and patient. It is from Mary McCarthy's *The Group*. After Dottie has had a contraceptive cap fitted this is what the doctor says to her: ' "Just a minute Dorothy," said the doctor, turning, and fixing her with her brilliant gaze, "Are there any questions?" ' A good approach; but listen to what happens:

Dottie hesitated; she wanted awfully, now that the ice was broken, to tell the doctor about Dick. But to Dottie's sympathetic eye, the doctor's lightly lined face looked tired. Moreover, she had other patients; there was still Kay waiting outside. And supposing the doctor, when she heard, should tell her to go back to the Vassar Club and pack and take the six o'clock train home and never see Dick again? Then the pessary would be wasted, and all would have been for nothing.

'Medical instruction,' said the doctor kindly, with a thoughtful look at Dottie, 'can often help the patient to the fullest sexual enjoyment. The young women who come to me, Dorothy, have the right to expect the deepest satisfaction from the sexual act.' Dottie scratched her jaw; the skin on her upper chest mottled. What she especially wanted to ask was something a doctor might know, above all, a married doctor. She had of course not confided in Kay the thing that was still troubling her: what did it mean if a man made love to you and didn't kiss you once, not even at the most thrilling moment? This was something not mentioned in the sex books, so far as Dottie knew, and perhaps it was too ordinary an occurrence for scientists to catalogue or perhaps there was some natural explanation, as she had thought before like hali or trench mouth. Or maybe he had taken a vow, like some people vowing never to shave or never to wash till a certain thing they wanted came about. But she could not get it out of her mind, and whenever she recalled it, not meaning to, she would flush all over, just as she was doing now. She was afraid down in her heart, that Dick was probably what Daddy called a 'wrong un'. And here was her chance to find out. But she could not, in this gleaming surgery, choose the words to ask. How would you put it in technical language? 'If the man fails to osculate?' Her dimple ruefully flashed; not even Kay could say such a thing. 'Is there anything abnormal . . .?' she began and then stared helplessly at the tall, impassible woman. 'If prior to the sexual act . . .' 'Yes?' encouraged the doctor. Dottie gave her throaty, scrupulous cough. 'It's terribly simple,' she apologized, 'but I can't seem to say it.' The doctor waited. 'Perhaps I can help you, Dorothy. Any techniques,' she began impressively, 'that give both partners pleasure are perfectly allowable and natural. There are no practices, oral or manual, that are wrong in love-making, as long as both partners enjoy them.' Goose flesh rose on Dottie; she knew, pretty well, what the doctor meant, and could not help wondering, with horror, if the doctor, as a married woman, practised what she preached. Her whole nature recoiled. 'Thank you, doctor,' she said quietly, cutting the topic off.[2]

I have read that as an example of a messianic doctor who has so urgently got a message to proclaim that she is totally insensitive to the real need of her patient even though she was trying desperately hard to meet it.

Now put just like that those are value-judgments. Let me simply say this by way of defence. Human suffering that you can't help hurts, and is therefore likely to be defended against. The patient who exposes one's ignorance, inadequacy, or one's neurotic conflicts, is at some level hated, resisted and is often even punished by the doctor.

Here, then, is a last and brief way of looking at this problem. Difficulties when they occur, when doctors regard their patients as difficult, or when patients regard their doctors as difficult, should be regarded as signals in their own right. It is not that they ought not to exist, but when they do happen what is the reason for them? They cry out in their own right for a diagnostic process and so to a learning process both for the doctor and for his patient when they are resolved. The feelings that are stirred up in you to make you hate your patient or to cry out when someone says 'Mr or Mrs So and So has come to see you', 'Oh heavens! No; tell them that I am out', or to look for some excuse, these feelings of difficulty should be taken as a situation in their own right from which we may learn why they are occurring and hence diminish them. And all that I have just been saying applies to the clergy as well.

2

In attempting to define precisely what is meant by a difficult patient I have reached the conclusion that all people are difficult patients and that it is only the degree of difficulty which varies from person to person. I begin from this viewpoint and shall try to define the factors which in my opinion transform the normal pleasant individual into a difficult patient – in much the same way that the same individual may be transformed into an anti-social monster when placed behind the driving wheel of a car. My remarks will be directed principally towards the hospital situation, although I hope they will also have relevance to the relationship between the patient and his GP.

The first factor which contributes towards the alienation of the individual – towards the creation of a difficult patient – is simply that the practice of medicine is a closed profession and not understood by the untrained mind. This, of course, is true of any profession, but no other impinges so directly on the individual, for in the practice of medicine the patient is subjected to the most intimate physical confrontation outside the privacy of marriage. In general practice this relationship can be developed gradually but in hospital it is often, by necessity, established rapidly on a purely arbitrary basis. In the extreme, the patient may be totally antagonistic from the beginning because of prejudice based on such simple things as the accent, physical appearance, or, more likely, the racial origin or sex of the doctor. Perhaps one day someone will give me a satisfactory explanation why the role of the female nurse is so completely accepted but there still remain elements of prejudice against the woman doctor. This prejudice is certainly much less intense than it was a few years ago as is well illustrated by a story, which I am sure is not apocryphal, of a husband and wife team in general practice. To the patients the man was always known simple as 'the doctor', while his wife was always referred to as 'the lady doctor'. History relates that one night in surgery the lady doctor poked in her head and said 'Next,please'. When no one moved after her second exhortation she pointed to a man sitting near the door and said, 'You'll do', to which he replied 'Oh, I am waiting for the doctor'. Quick as a flash she retorted 'What the hell do you think I am; a bloody vet?' History does not relate the further development of that relationship!

The second factor in the making of a difficult patient is fear of the unknown – an excellent basis on which to establish a difficult and unsatisfactory relationship. I think that unless the doctor knows his patient well he should always assume that apart from the simplest medical procedures such as taking the pulse or temperature, listening with a stethoscope, or taking blood pressure, all other medical manipulations are happening to the patient for the first time. It is a nerve-shattering experience to be in a situation where everyone from the trainee nurse upwards knows precisely what is to be done (and why) except the poor patient on which this standard routine procedure is to be perpetrated. At a time when every effort should be made to reassure the patient, this lack of information can increase his anxiety enormously. As a simple example take the case of the man who is admitted to hospital with a suspected heart condition. He is poked and prodded, tickled and hammered, interrogated often by a succession of people in increasing order of rank – then suddenly someone snaps out the efficient directive 'electrocardiogram'. Immediately the apprehension of the poor patient increases; he catches the phrase 'electro' and wonders if he will be able to withstand the inevitable electric shock; he then wonders if it involves sticking needles into various parts of his body. His mental torment increases until after several anxious minutes he finds that the procedure is quite painless, as a few wires are attached to him via suction cups. Of course the entire medical staff involved realized this but no one thought to tell the patient.

I am sure that most people can adjust themselves mentally to a time span of pain or discomfort if they are forewarned. Probably more difficult patients are created by lack of information than by any other single process. It is interesting to reflect that the success of such television soap-operas as *Dr Kildare* and *Emergency Ward 10* may be a direct outcome of the patients' desire to be taken into the confidence of their doctors in language which they can understand.

This brings me directly to my third point: the language with which the doctor attempts to communicate with his patient – if at all. This can vary from the one extreme of meaningless platitudes, 'Oh, yes, you'll be all right . . . don't worry', to a detailed discourse in technical language which leads rapidly to a glaze of incomprehension clouding the patient's eyes. Any profession, of course, needs its own language and jargon both for ease and accuracy of communication, but when talking to anyone outside the profession it is imperative to omit the technical language for simplicity and, if necessary, to sacrifice accuracy to ensure communication. There is a classic example which came to my attention some time ago which is worth giving to illustrate the use of language as a complete barrier to communication. It is taken from *The Lancet*:

> Experiments are described which demonstrate that in normal individuals the lowest concentration in which sucrose can be detected by means of gustation differs from the lowest concentration in which sucrose (in the amount employed) has to be ingested in order to produce a demonstrable decrease in olfactory acuity and a noteworthy conversion of sensations interpreted as a desire for food into sensations interpreted as satiation associated with the ingestion of food.

The English translation reads as follows: 'Experiments are described which show that a normal person can taste sugar in water in quantities not strong enough to interfere with his sense of smell or take away his appetite.'

The final point I wish to make concerns the impression inevitably given by medical doctors that their time is infinitely more valuable than that of the patient. This, of course, may be true, but it is at least diplomatic not to reveal the fact, and I am greatly encouraged by the recent trend to develop appointment systems as a matter of course in general practice. We have all met the doctor (or perhaps I have been unfortunate) who treats his patients to a quick pulse, a quick cough, a flick with the stethoscope, grunting incoherently all the while, scribbles a few indecipherable hieroglyphics on a prescription form and ushers the patient out, when the poor chap does not know if he is suffering from gout or bronchitis.

I realize that this question of time is extremely difficult but on the other hand I am convinced that a great deal of the doctor's time might be saved if he could spare a few minutes to talk in general terms to his patient, to attempt to find the person behind the symptoms, to understand his family situation, to know about his employment, for in many cases the cure may lie outside the individual himself.

You may have inferred from my arguments so far that I would place the main responsibility for the creation of difficult patients on the medical profession. If you have made this inference then you have interpreted my reasoning correctly. In most cases the patient is predominantly the passive partner in any relationship which is established and it is the prime responsibility of the doctor as the active partner to establish the level of communication relevant to the individual concerned. In thinking about the relationship between the medical profession in general and the public at large I realized that the nurses fill a very important intermediate role. I cannot speak highly enough of their quality, of their good humour and devotion to duty in often trying circumstances.

In most cases the patient and the family of the patient regards the nurse as an ally – as an interpreter between themselves and the more remote members of the medical team. In a sense the patient feels either explicitly, or implicitly, that as both he and the nurse are subjected to the authority of the doctor there is a link, to put it crudely, against the common enemy. If anyone doubts this thesis he has only to lie in a hospital bed and cooperate with the nursing staff in the mad scramble of activity to ensure that everything is in order for the Ward Round of Dr A. or Mr B. at 10 a.m. (of course he usually appears at 11 a.m., but this inconsistency cannot be relied on!). Perhaps it would be helpful if the doctors realized the strength of this bond between nurse and patient and attempted to exploit it (or rather use it) more to communicate indirectly with their patients.

In summary, then, it is my contention that difficult patients are in general not born but are created by certain shortcomings in the medical profession. They concern the ignorance of the patient over medical procedures; the real fear of the unknown; the patient's conviction that he is the only one who does not know what is going to happen; the use of either condescending platitudes or obscure medical jargon when the doctor attempts to talk to the patient; and the often inferred arrogance that the time of the doctor is always more valuable than that of the patient. It is surely important for the doctor to understand the whole person in order to treat him, and to develop a degree of confidence in their relationship. This clearly requires time to establish and a certain amount of judgment on the doctor's part to know how much he can safely tell the patient and in what language. In my opinion such effort would receive ample reward in the establishment of a true partnership between doctor and patient. For as a layman I feel that the element of the relationship must be one of partnership with the doctor ensuring that both partners are going in the same direction towards the common goal of good health. Without this co-operation we are likely to find ourselves in the position of the two men in a train compartment, one of whom asked the other, 'Where are you going?'; to which he replied 'London'. 'Oh,' said the first man, 'isn't British Rail wonderful? Here we are both on the same train: you are going to London and I'm going to Glasgow!'

NOTES

1. Michael Balint, *The Doctor, his Patient and the Illness*, Pitmans 1957
2. Mary McCarthy, *The Group*, Weidenfeld & Nicolson 1963, pp. 67f. Used by permission

D

7 Structures and Obstructions

1 *John Adair*
2 *R. W. Revans*

This chapter is composed of two addresses delivered at the 1968 Assembly of the Institute of Religion and Medicine at Oxford. The general title was 'Communication and Health'.

The first part is by Dr John Adair, who is not a medical doctor but a theologian and management consultant working with such diverse organizations as the Army, sections of industry, and the Church of England.

The second part is by Dr R. W. Revans, who also is not medically qualified but is a Research Fellow at the European Association of Management Training Centres in Brussels.

1

The thesis which I have been asked to discuss declares that there are structures within the church (as also in medicine) which block communication, and that to some extent these are obstructions which may be studied and perhaps eliminated.

I confess to having felt some reluctance in accepting this invitation. The trouble is that words like 'structure' and 'communication' have been bandied about so much that they are becoming void of meaning. Reflecting on his experiences at conferences in an entertaining broadcast entitled *A Sociologist fallen among Secular Theologians*,[1] Dr David Martin commented that at them the word 'structure' is as frequent as the word 'secular'. He went on to describe some of the familiar ingredients at such conferences: 'a fear of stereotypes and of images, and a sensitivity to the restricting power of roles, as well as to the rigidities of structure'. 'What is all the fuss about?' he asked. After all, roles will always crop up and reform movements will always become institutionalized. As for 'structure', what Max Weber called 'Rational Bureaucracy' is not only highly secular but also a necessary aspect of modern social organization. 'To object to it is to assert a radically religious drive which refuses to come to terms with the world. Genuine human existence and authentic personal life in modern communities depend on bureaucracy. Bureaucratic structure is an essential precondition of authenticity, not a barrier to it.'

In a sense David Martin has missed the point. The debate about structure in the church is not whether there should be one or not, but whether the present structure is a true one or not. And two of the criteria being advanced, are: first, the quantity and, more important, the quality of the communication which it permits vertically and horizontally; and secondly, the extent to which it creates an environment of health for those involved in it.

What do we mean by 'structure'? The *Concise Oxford Dictionary* offers this definition: 'Manner in which a building or organism or other complete whole is constructed, supporting framework or whole of the essential parts of something.' Note the use of the word 'whole' in the definition, which has strong links with our concept of health.

How can we understand or evaluate structure? Usually we do this in terms of purpose. The hand of a man or the wing of a bird are structures which excite our wonder when we see them at work, fulfilling their nature in action. All our appreciation of art and architecture stems from a similar survey of form in relation to purpose. Again at this point I should like to note a connection with health. With living organisms – biological and social – there may be a causal link between the proximity of a structure to its purpose and the concept of health. In other words a Rolls Royce car may structurally be highly appropriate to its purpose, but because it is never or rarely used for it, we may say that it becomes *majid*. Perhaps I should explain that this Arab word was once used to me in the middle of the Jordanian desert by my Bedouin Landrover driver while I was an officer in the Arab Legion. Opening the top of the silent bonnet he looked at the engine, and then at me. Shrugging his shoulders he said simply '*majid*!', which is a word used about camels with tummy trouble: it can best be translated as 'ill'. This kind of illness can assail us when we lack a purpose in life big enough to keep us healthy. A professor of medicine at Edinburgh, who made this last point to me, added that he once remembered saying absent-mindedly to his wife, while working single-handed in an Indian hospital during an epidemic, 'Don't worry, I am too busy be ill.'

Some organisms and organizations may be therefore structurally perfect, but wilting from a dislocation of purpose, while others may be vigorous in their life although anatomically imperfect. Although I am very interested in the theoretical anatomy of ecclesiastical organization and the articulation of its parts, I am much more concerned with the nexus between the structure as we have it now, with all its imperfections, and its purpose. It seems to me that this nexus or binding is weak. This in turn, to use St Paul's imagery, is the result of several organs of the body not fulfilling their proper function. Among these I should include the leadership of the church, for leaders exist to lead. Also I should add the theologians who have the responsibility of understanding and delivering to the leaders of the church the true ends to which they should guide its doing and its being. We can hardly blame the formal and informal communication channels – the nervous system – of the church. 'If the trumpet sounds uncertainly, who will answer the call?'

Does it matter? After all, it could be said, the churches are 'muddling through'. The men on the ground are doing a good job – comforting, baptizing, preaching and burying. Only the local and the personal matter, and there it all depends on the man. All that we ask of any ecclesiastical structure is that it serves up the right man in the right place and supports him financially. Then it is up to the individual. True, some clergymen have nervous breakdowns: the stress involved in a wide ignorance of purpose and in the lack of any completeness or wholeness in the ecclesiastical structure proves too much for their personalities; they cannot tolerate the ambiguities. But others, more creatively endowed, thrive and develop personalities like luxuriant and exotic orchids with no discipline of a clear purpose nor a fitting organization to keep them in check. Still others yet find a wholeness in relation to their own intuitive understanding of the gospel, and thereby give life to others.

It is not, however, these effects on the clergy and other professional ecclesiastics which most concern me here, but what might be called the 'sins of omission' in the church. If, as William Temple claimed, the church exists for the benefit of its non-members, we have a lot of explaining to do. Where are those local communities of Christians in which people are loved and valued not as instruments for human purposes, means to ends (even the ends of the local ecclesiastical or social structures), but as ends in themselves? In short, where are those communities in which love is doing its work?

At this point we may note how relatively little depends upon the personality and training of the clergyman: however good or bad he is he will possibly only affect the size and morale of his congregation 20% either way. He finds himself faced with a changing society, with sociological factors beyond his control, such as, for example, a large annual turnover of parishioners. The local church in such areas can take on a residual and elderly air, which does not attract the outsider. Moreover, the atmosphere of thought which people breathe today, which is no respecter of parish boundaries, adds to the general swing against the church. Counter-attacks on a diocesan or parochial scale, brilliant patrol actions and individual VC's do not disturb the general settled impression of the Receding Frontier (if I may borrow and mutilate a phrase of American historians), the erosion of the established cliffs, a yard a year. In such a situation it is not surprising that the clergy and laity look over their shoulders towards their leaders and their strategists, the theologians.

Does it matter? Yes, of course it does. People matter, and their growth into wholeness, their 'salvation', depends at each stage upon love. Love of God (in the double meaning of that phrase) is the Christian contribution to individuals, groups, society and to the world at large. Therefore it matters that the structure of the church should be corrected and brought into true in relation to its purpose. This in turn requires a much clearer understanding right down the line of that purpose, and why it is important. And that depends upon sound theological work and good leadership. But the fruits of advance will include social benefits: better communications, less obstruction and a more firmly based mental and physical health in the community as a whole.

2

Between 1952 and 1955 600 student nurses passed through the training schemes of the Royal Infirmary of a northern town and we were able to collect a complete health record of all of them; we knew when they were ill, and how long they stayed away in consequence. For us today, the interesting thing about these statistics is that this training scheme took the girls through a number of different hospitals; they all entered one preliminary training school and then they spent the next three years in moving between the main hospital and its subsidiary – or ancillary – hospitals. There were five or six such hospitals, including a maternity hospital, an eye hospital and a children's home.

When we came to analyse these statistics we found that every time the girls returned to one particular hospital they were more frequently sick than when they were in the other hospitals. Not only were they more frequently sick, but when they had fallen sick they stayed away longer, and the product of the more frequent sickness into the greater length of absence from work at this one hospital was about threefold the average over the other hospitals. In other words, the liability of a girl to be away ill while she was in one particular hospital was three times as great as when she was in any of the others, and since there were 600 girls in the sample this is, statistically, a highly significant result. Here we come right to the heart of the problem. Why does a dedicated creature like a nurse, under the surveillance both of doctors and of members of her own profession, fall sick more frequently in one hospital than in others in which she is training? As these girls were all near Manchester, we were able to hold frequent conversations with them, and especially to pursue this remarkable effect. We did not in fact tell them that this was what we were interested in; we merely encouraged them to talk about their experiences as nurses in training. It very soon became clear that the difference which they saw between the hospital in which they were frequently sick and the other hospitals was that in the latter they could get answers to the questions which they put. Nor was that all. After we had begun to know them better they explained that in these hospitals (that is, the ones where they were seldom ill) they were even helped to frame the questions which otherwise they would not have known how to put. In a situation of confusion, as in a hospital ward, it is no good saying to a young student nurse, 'Well, you've got a tongue in your head, haven't you?' Of course she has, but if she is so confused about her task that she cannot find the words to express herself, having a tongue in her head will not be of the slightest use to her. One can put into words only ideas that are already forming themselves.

What is the significance of this? It is quite simple. In the hospital in which it is not recognized that the nurse needs help to put questions when she is confused, her confusion is never allayed; on the contrary, anxiety is generated and she falls ill. It is not suggested that

the doctors and nurses in the traumatic hospital were more unkind
or uncharitable than those in the other hospitals; they may have
been more busy, engaged on all kinds of highly complicated things,
or possibly that particular hospital was full of professors – whose
absorptions in their own affairs always create complications. But the
most significant point is that, in the hospital where the girls were so
frequently sick, the persons in authority seemed unaware of the
impact they were having on their subordinates. Here I might quote
from St Paul's Epistle to the Galatians, 6.2,3: 'For if a man think
himself to be something, when he is nothing, he deceiveth himself.
But let every man prove his own work and then shall he have re-
joicing in himself alone and not in another.' Perhaps the Jacobean
English seems a little obscure, but what it means is this: if you
think you are somebody very important, and you go through life
always with this thought in your head, then you remain unaware of
the impact you are making on other people and you have no genuine
opportunity to prove – or test – your own work. In particular you
cannot be communicated with, and thus cannot learn where you
stand. You have an unrealistic self-image, to use the jargon of a
modern psychologist. When this is the misfortune of those at the top
of the hospital, all within it must share the same myopia. If father
cannot learn, then all the family remain in the dark. You must all
know the reference of Ecclesiasticus, 10.2: 'As the judge of the
people is himself, so are his officers; and what manner of man the
ruler of the city is, so are all they that inhabit therein.' You may
have heard it in more colloquial terms: 'There are no bad soldiers,
only bad generals' or, even, 'Fish goes rotten from the head.'

Leaving the particular group of hospitals where the 600 girls were
training, and looking at a sample of other acute general hospitals, we
discovered that these institutions differed significantly in the clarity
of their internal communication systems. Any communication
begins and ends in the consciousness of the human being; it is not, as
many people imagine, merely a matter of telephone lines or inputs
to computers or messengers running around carrying pieces of
paper – this is a very incomplete view, indeed. We must think of the
consciousness of the people who either emit the messages or receive
them. We must also be aware of their self-consciousness, or of their
self-awareness. What is the amount of meaning that is transmitted
between people when they talk to each other? This meaning can be
obscured for many different reasons: in the first place because one of

the persons may never have 'proved his work'; he may be unaware of the impact he is making upon other people; he may be so unaware that he terrifies his subordinates and they become afraid to ask him questions. This may be one reason. Or it may be that the man is so busy with details that he loses his sense of priorities; he is trying to deal decisively with all kinds of unimportant matters rather than trying to define the important ones. There may be many reasons why the demands made upon persons working together cannot be adequately met, but almost invariably one is lack of intelligible communication between them.

Now this is a highly practical problem. What can we do about it? . . . If we pursue these studies in other fields, whether in coal-mines or factories, or even secondary-modern schools, we find very similar problems. We find also, in studying children in a school classroom, that different teachers have very different perceptions of their role *vis-à-vis* children. Some teachers believe it is their job to keep order, which means to suppress voluntary communication from the children. Other teachers, risking the disapproval of the inspectors and the directors of education (whose first concern is to avoid trouble), run their classes like a bear garden, with the children free to interrupt at any time and pose any relevant question they like. The test of the teacher is his ability to reject the irrelevant. It is possible to show that it is in the bear garden of relevant interruption that children learn, because the teacher has a chance of finding out what it is that they do not understand, after they are given an opportunity to communicate it. If the child cannot communicate, or is prevented from expressing his doubt at the time he has it, there is no meaningful communication between the two, and thus no learning, either by child or by teacher. In the hospital, too, the doctor who listens to the nurse both helps her to learn and improves his own knowledge of what is going on among his patients. It can be shown that doctors who express an awareness of their own needs to learn are those most conscious of the problems of their staff. And indifference to the needs of others is correlated with a satisfaction about the self.

Our problem is what, in terms of practical action, we can do to improve communications. And here I would like to quote again, from Luke 17.20: 'And when they demanded of him when the kingdom of heaven should come he answered them and said "The kingdom of heaven cometh not by outward show [some authorities translate it 'by observation'], neither shall ye say 'Lo, here' nor 'Lo, there' [which means 'It's no good looking for it here; it's no good looking for it there']; for, behold, the kingdom of heaven is within you.'' This is exactly the problem of communication in industry. We are not going to improve communications between human beings merely by feeding information into computers, saying 'Lo, it's over there, in a system of integrated data processing', nor 'Lo, it's over here, with new reporting rules for the foremen', nor 'Lo, it's at the business school, with its seminars to clarify the (supposed) relations between line and staff. . . .' We are going to improve communications only when people realize that the kingdom of God is within themselves, as the origins and destinations of the messages; in other words, the key is to be found in our internal attitudes towards others, in our respect for others, in our willingness to listen to what other people are trying to say to us, and in the effort we make to understand them. At the moment the French, of course, seem concerned about this, and are even talking a great deal about keener understanding and shared responsibility by participation; nevertheless, they are not very clear about what they mean. But, faced with practical necessities, the French seldom are clear, although they have a reputation for being logical. What will actually happen if and when the President seeks to build participation in the factories I do not know; I shall be interested to see. But from the various universities in Europe with whom I am working, we are attempting to involve persons in industry in the examination of the day-to-day transmission of meaning from one person to another. Our text is from I Corinthians 8.1, 2: 'Now as touching things offered unto idols, we know that we all have knowledge. Knowledge puffeth up, but charity edifieth.' The need is not for more technical communication but for more understanding, or charity, to use the biblical term, of relationships between persons. We should lift this text from the New Testament and apply it to the affairs of an oil refinery or a coal-mine or a factory. It is not lack of knowledge that promotes strikes, but lack of wisdom.

We have already tried to stress the notion of the self-image, in groups of factories and hospitals, and some here may have heard about the consortium of ten hospitals in London, which recognized the need for improving their internal communications by setting out to clarify the perceptions of the staff about who they were and what they meant to others. One can do nothing, in any field, not only in

communications, for anybody unless he first recognizes the need for
something to be done; you cannot cure a man of the drink unless he
wants to be cured of the drink; there must be some predisposing
motivation to do something about role perceptions, and it must
preferably be the senior person in the hospital or the factory – the
ruler of the city of Ecclesiasticus – who is motivated to make the
institution more effective. Normal persons will not improve their
communications, either in hospitals or factories or pits, merely by
listening to lectures by professors about the virtues of doing so,
although once motivated, the second step in effective action is to
identify themselves with those giving them advice; without confidence in your adviser you are wasting your time and his as well.
In my view, the best persons to perceive the shortcomings of one
hospital are those from other hospitals who have been trained to
pose the discriminating questions. You may well say that this is a
case of the blind leading the blind, or of the man with the beam in his
eye offering to pluck the mote from the eye of another, but this is
not so. A surgeon who suspects that the progress of patients through
his operating theatre is not as effective as it might be is not going to
listen to advice from a professor not medically qualified. But deeds
may change him where words but cause resentment. He might,
that is, learn something from a practical exercise conducted with
another surgeon, especially a surgeon who does not share his
responsibility for the situation in that particular operating theatre.

Our strategy was this: to get the senior staffs of ten hospitals
together and invite them to look into what is going on in each
other's dominions. We find that by encouraging people of the same
rank to discuss their problems, with a little judicious advice upon
how to programme their discussions, it is possible suddenly to make
them conscious that they may not, after all, be as closely in contact
with other persons – nor with their own objectives – as they ought to
be. We also confirm the text of Ecclesiasticus, for there is a very
high correlation between the improvement of role relations and the
enthusiasm shown by the senior staff to get personally involved in
the efforts to improve them. As one practical result of this experiment, the Royal College of Physicians is holding a national meeting
to which nearly 300 consultants are coming, and they are going to
discuss this very question, that is, their perception of themselves
vis-à-vis other people in their hospitals. Who might they think they
are? Who do any of us think we are? Why do we say the things we

do? Why, in particular, do we say things that we know to be untrue? Why do we stop others from saying things we know to be true – unless, of course, we earn our livings, like public relations officers, by deliberately and professionally confounding what we know to be the truth? And even then do we recognize that a policy of deceiving others always ends as a means of deceiving ourselves? Do we ever reflect upon such questions?

We have been able to devise survey instruments which encourage our doctors to reveal who, in fact, they think they are. We have been experimenting in this way, led by some of the consultants in our consortium of ten hospitals, and the result of the research stands out with a clarity so luminous that even doctors are interested in it. It shows that the doctor who is not particularly sensitive to his need to profit from his clinical experiences, or who is not aware that every case he handles might be teaching him something, is the doctor who is not much concerned with the problems and tribulations of the people with whom he works. The man who cannot interpret the events that crowd in on him as lessons – indeed, the only lessons – that should be teaching him something, making him, if you like, a more aware doctor, is the man unconcerned with the difficulties of the institution around him, content to tolerate or even to defend its inefficiencies.

We find this to be a general result: it appears among managers of breweries in Denmark, managers of glass factories in Belgium. The man who, in the words of St Paul, does not prove his own work, and so is unaware of how his daily experience should be enriching his perception of himself, is at the same time the man who cannot see that the hospital or factory in which he works is in need of help to become a better institution. To some extent this, of course, is an institutional influence and has social implications; some hospitals, as total institutions, are socially aware, and encourage their individual members to become personally aware. It is possible to compare among themselves not only different hospitals but different factories or different schools (among those hospitals in which the girls do not go sick and those in which they do, among the factories always on strike and those which are not, among the universities that have to call in the police and those that stick to philosophy) and to say how much of their differences, one from another, can be attributed to purely organizational factors, how much to purely informational factors, and how much is due to their self-awareness, the perception of their roles *vis-à-vis* other people. The third is the most important single influence and it is thus our task in management education to increase the self-awareness of our managers. In a complex world such as the one we are now living in, the need is for understanding the relevance of one's own place in the situation one is trying to influence. It is this sensitivity to how the persons with whom you are working interpret what you are saying, or trying to say, that is important. In my view, this is a subject essentially for the theologian. The art of listening, of concentrating the attention, is helpful, but not enough. I must convince my speaker that I respect him enough to want to know what he is trying to say to me. Since every minute I spend in listening to him is gone for good, I am in fact offering him the most precious resource I have. It is a noble thing voluntarily to offer one's time to another out of a simple respect for him as a person. (It is more common, alas, to find that the time offered to others is directly proportional to an estimate of how useful they might be.) Thus, although you may say that identification with others is a subject for the psychiatrist, to identify and to assess the ultimate value-system governing the depth of involvement seems to me a religious question.

Since I am neither theologian nor psychiatrist, but only a statistician, I am entitled to say that, given a choice between a psychiatrist and a theologian as to which would help me make most progress, I would choose the theologian. My own trade helps me define the crucial differences between the good and the poor hospitals; the psychiatrist tells me of the operational effects of stress and of identification, and with his help, and that of the management scientist, we can devise projects for illuminating the effects that we have on each other, and, in particular, the effects that seniors have upon their juniors. But all this, though it may earn us our daily bread and even move an occasional university to offer us their honorary degree, is only to use the knowledge that St Paul recognizes to puff us up. Whence comes the charity that alone can edify? For, as I have reason to know, something more is needed to run our hospitals than knowledge. Even the universities can no longer subsist on a diet of pure intellectualism; their problems will not be solved by subtlety of dialectic nor by profusion of facilities. We must learn to respect persons as well as techniques. The debatable issue is the practical means of so learning. What I am sure of is that much is possible if we believe the pursuit of such self-understanding to be worthwhile. But about the source of these beliefs and values I am not qualified to speak. This task is for the theologian.

NOTE

1. *The Listener*, 25 April 1968

8 Good News and Bad News

1 David Jenkins
2 Louis Marteau

This chapter is composed of two addresses delivered at the 1968 Assembly of the Institute of Religion and Medicine at Oxford, when the general theme was 'Communication and Health'.

The first part is by Canon David Jenkins, who was then Fellow and Chaplain of The Queen's College, Oxford. In 1969 he moved to Switzerland to direct the World Council of Churches' '*Humanum* Project' – the search for an answer to the question, 'What constitutes a human being?'

The second part is by the Reverend Louis Marteau, who is Roman Catholic Chaplain at the London Hospital.

1

In facing the question 'Should the doctor tell?' and its equivalents, two principles strike me as being relevant. The first principle is that the primary question is not whether the news is good or bad but whether it is true, and the second principle is that every person is as such (i.e. as a person) entitled to know the truth. Two very obvious principles, but it seems to me all the more necessary to be clear about them because, as far as I can judge, they nearly always have to be so acutely modified in practice that they rapidly become obscured and forgotten. This applies not only in what tend to be called 'clinical' situations but in a variety of situations in which persons for various reasons are to some extent authority figures and are expected to give advice or convey information and so on. The particularities of those situations *always* modify one's applications precisely because the application is such a difficult matter. It is almost certain (quite certain?) that in acting we obscure our principles up to a point. Hence we have to start this type of discussion by establishing and repeating the obvious.

The first principle, then, is that the primary question is not whether the news is good or bad, but whether it is true; by which I mean, without getting involved in too great a debate about the nature of truth, does it correspond with reality, actuality, probability. I think I discern a certain tendency to dodge one's responsibilities for conveying the actualities of a situation on the grounds that it is only probable, and not certain. In discussions about 'Should the doctor tell?' or 'What should the clergyman say?' there is need to be careful not to hide behind what I would call improbable evaluations of probability.

In using this phrase I have in mind a difficult situation about good news and bad news, in which even the most 'committed unbeliever' is prepared to fall back on the notion of miracles. ('Miracles do happen, so we cannot be quite sure, so there is no need to tell. . . .') That is what I call an improbable evaluation of probability. The probable evaluation of probabilities is 'This is what is bound to happen.' It is quite possible that a wrong judgment is being made, but the person concerned is in the position that he is because of his competence, responsibility and experience. Therefore his judgment of what is probable must be taken as being the judgment which is probable and on which one has to act. These improbable judgments of probability are never made when the subject is something which is good or found easy to do. Then one acts upon a normal judgment of probability, and so one must in 'bad' situations.

Therefore, with regard to the question 'Is it true?', I simply mean does it correspond to what is probably the truth, the reality, the actuality, using a normal evaluation of probability. This approach has a theological basis. For the Christian the question of truth, the question of reality, is in fact the crucial and basic one because God is in reality. He is nowhere else. Most of us tend to spend most of the time endeavouring to find God in what I have come more and more to call the 'neither here nor there' – that is to say not in the transcendent reality which is God nor in the present reality which is now. But it is quite clear theologically speaking, as it is practically speaking, that God is in reality – to be met with only in and through reality – what actually is, what is actually happening, what is actually going on.

The theological doctrines which support this view are those of Creation, Incarnation and Redemption, but there is no space to expand this. It is the Christian belief that God is responsible for reality (Creation), that God is capable of being involved in reality (Incarnation), and that God can make Heaven out of a hell of a mess (Redemption). This would be the 'doctrinal' way of making the point that the one place where the believer in God has got to be is 'in reality'. A more 'evangelical' way of stating the same thing would be simply to refer to Jesus Christ, the cross, the resurrection, as the pattern of things which is the pattern of producing worthwhileness in reality. Therefore I deduce theologically the principle that the basic question always is – 'What reality is there to come to terms with?' Because of the gospel there is always a hopeful possibility here. This, therefore, leads me on to make the formulation that, in fact, real news is good news and false news is bad news. Such would seem to me to be the implications of Christian faith. Certainly it seems quite clear that Christians have a realistic faith which has to be put to the test of reality and which sees reality as the place where it therefore follows that real news is good news and that false news is bad news, and this is what has to be borne in mind when one faces up to a situation.

My second principle is this. Every person as such is entitled to know the truth. Here I think that those of us who find ourselves in authority situations need to consider that what I might call the condescension of the unsure authoritarian is a very horrid thing. It is also a very frequent thing. We must be crystal clear that it cannot be the case that any person is an inferior being. Further, you cannot take ultimate responsibility for him or her, whoever you are. All this talk about *my* patients, *my* flock, or *my* clients is dangerously close to blasphemy. No amount of medical ethics or social work ethics or even psychotherapeutic ethics must obscure this fact, because ethics which obscure this fact are not ethics but are actually sins.

I feel bound to say that the more experience I have the more I come to the conclusion that if I want a professional man in any sphere, while his professional qualifications must be satisfactory, the really important criterion for choosing him is his humility. Without humility he is liable to do a great deal of damage. Consequently, all of us – not only medical men but also ministers, priests and the rest – have to be very clear that to withhold what is a personal entitlement is a very grave thing; indeed, it is the ultimately grave thing if you care for persons.

Nevertheless, a final qualification must be made. It is also clear

that persons are very often not persons enough to bear their entitlement. Indeed, I think this applies to all of us. I am always troubled
by talk of 'getting what one is entitled to'. Personally, I am very
afraid that some Commission or other will come along and give me
what I am entitled to! My great reason for putting my hope in God
is that I believe he has persuaded me that he is certainly not going to
give me what I am entitled to. In any case, it does seem sufficiently
clear that persons cannot necessarily bear that to which they are
entitled. Therefore, I would say in closing that it does not follow
from my two principles that the practical rule is – always tell the
whole truth. I am aware that to suggest that you may not have to
face persons with the whole truth is to beg all sorts of questions
because 'unwhole truth' tends to be false. We certainly have complications here but I fear we cannot escape the fact there are no
general rules in personal situations. Being personal is far too responsible a thing for that. We cannot take refuge in general rules.

I have been talking about general principles which have to be
applied in particular circumstances, and my qualification may be
thought to have destroyed the whole value of this general statement.
Nevertheless, I believe that the sort of thing that would follow from a
serious and sustained facing up to my two principles would be as
follows. Firstly, much more would be told to many more people. I
believe that there is a good deal of withholding of both good news
and bad news because of what is involved if you actually commit
yourself to the persons involved sufficiently to tell it to them. For
this means that you get involved in the reality of the situation rather
than in the situation at one remove by virtue of some sort of clinical
or psychiatric relationship. Such a relationship one has to have
because one cannot deal directly with more than so many people.
Nevertheless serving persons does demand maturity beyond such a
relationship and I think on the whole it would follow that much more
would be told to many more people.

Secondly, we should all have to look for, and would, I am sure,
certainly receive, much more of what I can only call 'grace' – grace
to be much more really with people in the realities of their situations,
whether they were receiving good news or facing bad news. Surely
it is this being in the realities of the situation with people which
seems to me to make the real demand and provide the basic criterion
with regard to the telling of good news or bad news.

2

I see this business of 'communicating' and 'communicator' as being vital in so far as it highlights the primary role of the priest, a constant subject of discussion. He is a communicator in the fullest sense of the word. Primarily we have the gospel, which is the good news. The communication of the gospel is the object of preaching and of the daily routine of pastoral work. It is the good news into which all events are taken up, absorbed and elevated by the consideration of them in the framework of the love of God, which is redemption.

Thus the primary purpose of the priest is one of communicating. In some disciplines this is added to by its second form, the sacramental communication. This in a way underlines the first in so far as it is a visible outward sign of this communication acted out by the people concerned, emphasizing and re-establishing the validity and the reality of it. Communication begins in the mind of the communicator and ends in the mind of the recipient, and the sacramental communication with God begins in the mind of God and ends in the soul of the recipient: all the liturgical paraphernalia which surround it are merely there to open out each individual in turn to the fullness of the power of that communication. These communications contain, always, both the good and the bad. The bad is contained in the good. Light and shade go together. In baptism the sign is the sign of death, of death with Christ and resurrection with Christ as a new person. In the eucharist, the memorial of the sacrifice and the expectancy of the eucharistic meal of love with Christ run together with the sacrifice contained in the eucharistic thanksgiving, banquet of the good news. I think this too needs emphasizing in the sacrament of matrimony, where the giving of each individual, the renunciation in some sense of their own ideologies, their own way of life, their individual freedom to one another is only resurrected in the acceptance of it by the other person, and in the acceptance of the other person's giving. These two things run constantly in the theme of Christian thought. There can be in some sense no good news which does not contain the bad; and the bad is only the obverse of the good. The final communication of God was in Christ and was a communication of himself as a full person – a full, feeling, emoting human being. His answer to the problem of life was not a catch-phrase, was no clarion call, was no political and final solution to every single problem. His answer was the living out of the bad in the concept of the good; to suffer all that man could suffer, to render himself open to all physical and emotional problems that man could experience, even to final abandonment by God, and to do this in demonstration of the acceptance of man by God in total love.

This sort of thing is underlined to me very strongly in the pastoral situation. I remember a girl of about seventeen who was dying of cancer, a cancer in one shoulder that was like a rugby ball. It was getting so bad that we were frightened that the arm would disarticulate before she died. She even picked out bits of bone when the nurse did the dressings. This lassie had a bad family background. Mother and father were at loggerheads with each other, her boy friend walked out on her, she was alone, she was abandoned. She said she had prayed and prayed and she felt that God did not listen to her. So I said to her, 'Well, say it then: tell him he's abandoned you'. Eventually she did. Then I said to her, 'Now you're with Christ on the cross: that's what he said', and she suddenly got the message. She got it a bit queerly and I am not sure whether the theologians present would agree with her final summation which was, 'I see what I must do now; I must forget God and be with Christ.' But it was not the time for theological disputation. The idea was there and the completeness of the situation was there. She changed from that time.

In this sort of situation what answer could there be except this communication of Christ in his totality? The priest is in some sense the continuation of his incarnation. The communication of the good news has got to be personalized, humanized. The communication must be one of flesh and blood, not merely of words. The understanding must be a living entity, within the framework of a human relationship. It can only take place in the situation of a human relationship. This human relationship enables us to work within the limits of the understanding or the capability of acceptance of each separate individual. This means that the communicator needs intense sensitivity to each individual in each relationship. This is the place of wisdom.

It is a basic relationship, a relationship where every man is equal. It goes beyond and below patterns and roles, a great many of which are forced upon us by the culture in which we live. All the world is a stage and all the men and women merely actors. And we are dealing with them not as kings and princes or serving maids, but as actors, and as actors each one is equal.

It is not just a simple communication; it is not just a simple message. The relationship and the message have to be catalytic. They produce some sort of result, or rather, allow some sort of change to take place, a change which will affect both parties in the relationship.

As Canon Jenkins said earlier, the communication must be 'true'. I should like to put communication and health together, health and wholeness. The communication must be healthy. I do not know if we altogether know what truth is, but I think we have a slight idea of what healthy communication is, a wholeness of communication. It must be all inclusive against the whole pattern of life, with a depth of vision which includes the total vision of human life in God's providence. And therefore although one is communicating one part it must be in the sense of the whole. There must be the wholeness about the individual communication. One is not passing concepts, and certainly not passing words. Words are instruments which can be played with, while concepts are cold intellectual ideas. One is making a human communication to a human being, which means that, in effect, the person to whom one is communicating must react in a human fashion in the same way to that particular item as it exists within the communicator. The reaction must be, in due proportion, the same as the reaction to the facts formed within the communicator. Then only has the communication reached its perfection.

The perspective that one is trying to give has to create the same perspective in the person to whom one is communicating. This again requires sensitivity and understanding, as to the level at which the other person can accept it, and thus in what way one puts it over.

Truth, yes. This is one of our big difficulties. There has been so much covering up of the bad, not being able to speak about the bad, that now people no longer react to truth when they hear it. I remember a patient who had his leg amputated. He gradually went down and down, although the doctor could find no medical reason for his deterioration. In spite of this it was becoming increasingly obvious that he was dying. I asked him, 'Are you expecting to die?' He said 'Yes'. I said, 'Well it looks as if you're going to, but the only reason you're going to is you've decided to. There's no physical reason why you should, but you certainly will because you have decided that that's what's going to happen. Why have you decided that you are going to die?' And he told me. The doctor had told two other men in the ward who'd had amputations that they were perfectly all right and would be out in a few weeks. Both died. The doctor said exactly the same thing to him: therefore he had been told he was going to die. It is very difficult when one is covering up on one side to be able to tell the wholeness of truth on any other.

In the hospital the situation of the patient becomes somewhat complicated in the question of communicating. There is a natural regression to childhood, and I think, a rightful regression. It is very ignominious for an adult to have to suffer the child-like attentions of the nurse while they are still in an adult frame of mind, such as being bathed, powdered, oiled and patted. They need to be allowed to regress to some extent, to suffer such ignominies. And one has to make a certain allowance for the fact that this person has regressed in the way one is communicating to him. On the other hand there are certain times when the communication is so important that they must be drawn out of the child pattern and brought back into an adult situation in order to face an adult truth.

I remember a fellow who was determined to take his discharge. He was suffering from a very bad lung condition and I doubted very much whether he would get to the end of the staircase in the state he was in. Everybody was worried about this but it was not until I walked up to him and saw him in my mind standing up in his trousers and jacket, a full-size man of six foot four, that I could then say to him, 'If you want to take your discharge, take it, but you're going to have to sign a chitty so that the coroner will excuse the hospital of any responsibility. And be a pal, turn left as you go out the hospital; 200 yards down the road is an undertakers. Get things organized and save the family a lot of trouble.' This is the sort of communication I would make with a man in full possession of himself as an adult. He turned back and said, 'Is that how I am?' I said, 'Well, I'm not playing around with you'. He said, 'Right: well I'll stay in', and that was that. He later went out considerably better.

I think that there are times when one has to try in this communicating to bring the patient back into adult form. I go round the wards and I accept their regressed state. I try to assist them to 'a purposeful expression of negative feelings', as it says in the textbooks, to grumble, in other words, so that I can discover from them where communication has broken down, where they are having problems, and perhaps by pouring a little oil on the water and getting things a little more organized, solve simple problems. But then, having allowed this for a period, I begin to build them back again to adults before leaving. Building them back into adults becomes even more vital when they are looking towards discharge. And here, by talking to the women about their children, to the men about their jobs, you begin to get them back into an adult situation where they can talk about their responsibilities and see themselves as a responsible person.

I remember a little fellow, an Italian, who was regressing very badly. He had not in fact got very long to live, but he was going down much faster than he ought and had become completely depressed, and was becoming very isolated from the ward situation. He was a sculptor and made tombstones and statues for cemeteries. I started chatting to him about this. 'Tell me about it. How long would it take you to do one of these things?' And he said, 'Well, you know, tell me what you want and I'll tell you how long it takes. I work on the clock; it's a business. You want a lily, two hours for a lily. I watch the clock, two hours later – a lily. I'm no Michelangelo: that's a lily, two hours.' He got so worked up about this that he came out of his depression and within four or five days he was away. It drew him out of his isolation, and once again replaced him as a craftsman doing a crafty job.

One interesting thing to observe in a hospital like mine, a general hospital, with one psychiatric unit, is the different attitudes which exist towards patients. The general patient coming in, a man possibly of some standing, with the small whitlow that we have heard about before, is immediately stripped and his clothes are whipped off to the far end of the establishment; he is thrown into bed; confined; and so regresse into childhood. He may not leave the ward even for an instant without an attendant nurse. If he goes to X-ray, a porter must convoy him. If he is to go to the chapel, then somebody must go up and convoy him. Next door is the psychiatric ward where the patient is not allowed to go to bed, not allowed to take off his clothes (they sometimes do but they are not supposed to). They are not allowed to be escorted to X-ray or to occupational therapy if they are capable of going on their own. In fact, on Sundays, if I have a catholic patient in a general ward who wants to go to Mass I have to get a psychiatric patient to accompany him!

The staff communications that go on in these two separate wards are again fascinating and the dynamics of them interesting to watch.

The nurse who for the first six months of her life in this establishment has been following the traditions of Florence Nightingale and Edith Cavell, lining up in the morning, having herself inspected and being told off as to her duties and silently paraded around the ward and despatched to her coffee break and so on, arrives in the psychiatric ward to discover a sister and staff nurse dressed in mufti sitting down to a cup of coffee saying, 'Do join us. What's your Christian name? Have a cigarette. How do you feel this morning?' After three months of this, the nurse is oriented slightly differently towards her general set-up, goes back on to another ward where she is once more lined up and marked off. How long this can continue before the two systems have an effect on each other, one wonders. Certainly the sister on a ward situation in the psychiatric block is concerned totally with communication. She sees the importance of the nurse being allowed to communicate to her how she feels in herself, her relationships with the patients, and the feelings of the patients. The sister's role is more vital in terms of communication.

In considering communicating, we tend to get terribly bound up in the problems of life and death. I do not think that hospitals tend to be places where life and death are really the biggest problem. 'I've been saving lives all day', the junior houseman will say as we gather round the bar. In point of fact there are very few times he has been saving lives. Most of the time he is dealing with a much lower level of function. But the communications are worse down at that lower level than anything at the top. If somebody is dying everybody asks the same question, 'Who's going to tell him? How are they going to tell him? What are we going to do?' This can go on for a week. No, it is right at the bottom level that the real trouble occurs. I remember a young Maltese girl – four months pregnant – very worried, terribly disturbed, screaming to go home. She had a slight heart murmur so they wanted to keep her there, but she was so upset no one could control her. I walked over to the lassie and said, 'Did your mother ever tell you anything about having babies?' And she said 'No' – as simple as that. She thought she had a cancer growing in her stomach because she did not know where babies came from. This is where it all started, a simple straightforward communication. I asked the sister to go and take her some pictures and talk to her for a bit.

But it is right down at this level of communicating that things tend to go wrong. Patients are pushed off to one place or another; people descend upon them with all sorts of machinery; all sorts of procedures go on, and time and time again they are not told; not told because the person does not want to tell them what they are looking for in case it is not there. But at least they could explain what they are looking *at*, if they could not explain what they are looking *for*. The level of communication on the small things tends to be bad, and this is where so much trouble comes up. There are the obvious gaffs that go on. It is unfortunate in medical terminology that every miscarriage is an abortion, and young girls who wanted a child and have unfortunately had a miscarriage hear themselves referred to as 'the abortion in bed four' by accident. This causes no end of pain and unnecessary misery.

I think that the top level communications are not so bad, but this may not be so right down at the bottom level. Here again I can come back to considering the priest in his role of communicator, the human communicator with a small 'c'. His relationships on a human level with the staff in the hospital setting – the fact that in the sight of the patient the doctor and the chaplain nod at each other is seen as an externalized communication, and sometimes bridges a gap in the patients' minds between themselves and the doctor. Normally the priest is not the person they are frightened of; the doctor is. If the priest shows he is frightened of the doctor too when he walks in the ward, and skids out as if the Big White Chief were on his rounds, then this can be feeding fear into the patients. He has got to be able to break through this barrier of role, and forget role and forget the act, and get down to the actor. He has not only to bridge the gap but at the same time he has to avoid being cast with any of the acting roles, not becoming part of the doctor class and so making a gap between himself and the patients.

I have been fascinated by this subject of 'Communications and Health', wondering whether it was theologically even deeper than one thought. Could it link up with the communications being lost with God in original sin (however one defines it), and ill-health coming in, and even death? Is not communication both with God and with man the whole background and basis of our work in the Christian ideology?

9 Dimensions of Death

Cicely Saunders

Dr Cicely Saunders trained both as a nurse and a social worker, and had some experience as a patient, before her interest in the needs of dying patients led her to read medicine. She qualified in 1957 and was able to take up a Research Fellowship, working among patients with terminal malignant disease at St Joseph's Hospice. During seven years' work there, and in the planning of St Christopher's Hospice which opened in 1967 and of which she is Founder Member and Medical Director, the importance of teaching in this area became an increasing preoccupation.

The chapter that follows was a talk commissioned by the Religious Department of the BBC European Services for what is known in Germany as 'The Day of the Dead'. It has been twice broadcast in its German translation on the European network.

I have known many dying patients and their families while I have been working as a doctor and as a nurse, but what I will try to say about death and dying comes above all from my own personal experience. However close you may come to a patient, however much they may become real friends (and with many of the very ill this happens), yet it is from personal impact of bereavement that one can readily speak of such things. All the same, my work has had an effect upon my own thoughts and feelings, above all, giving the comfort of knowing that even in loneliness itself we belong with an infinite number of others who have similar problems to face. Even as we remember and mourn our own unique and irreplaceable one we are reminded that the same kind of pain is felt by countless others and that we are not alone.

This kinship stretches back in time as well as across space. From the moment when a little hoard of flints was placed in the grave of early man, the human race has laid down its dead in grief. And it has done so with the hope that somehow this was not the end, and that somewhere those flints would be needed.

Dying may be hard; it may mean diminishing faculties and the loss of independence; it may bring weakness and suffering, or the sudden, harsh end of all that concerned one in this world. But this is not all that I see as I walk round our wards today, as I remember countless others, among them some most near to me. There is another dimension, which by its existence alters the whole character of dying. We believe this as we see that death itself is something quite distinct from the process of dying and that just as many people make it the greatest achievement of this part of their lives, so they show us truths beyond the purely material world.

One of my greatest friends was a girl who was only forty years old when she died. For the first years I remember she gradually became paralyzed and blind and for the last three years was totally without sight and almost without any movement at all. Many of us came to be her friends, but it was another patient who best summed up what one saw in her as she lived on in the midst of this slow dying of her body. As she came away from her bedside one afternoon this patient said to us, 'The incredible thing is, you don't even feel sorry for her: she is *so* alive.' Her dying had become the very means of her growth, for we learnt from her husband that her intense aliveness, gaiety and interest in other people had developed during her illness. Always we remember her laughter, made more vivid by the occasional tears that showed us how much this cost her. The less her body could do the more her spirit shone, in love and amusement and a clear-sighted wisdom concerning life and those she met. Body and mind are linked indissolubly but they are of much less account than the spirit whose purposes they serve. That is not only unique and irreplaceable; it is also indestructible, stronger even than the light and energy of the star which streams across the universe millions of years after its source has ceased to exist.

When this girl died she left something that goes on living and developing in the life of her husband, her friends, and in the foundation now built for patients such as herself. While she was ill she found faith in God, reaching out trustfully at first to what she saw dimly as true and finding that this constantly became clearer, more secure and more personal. She had many advantages: a husband who never let her down, and so many new friends that she once described God's dealings with her, 'He sends me people.' Such achievement in dying itself is not unique, nor totally dependent on those around the patient. Many of us can look back and say firmly of those we have lost, however hard and lonely their path may have seemed, that it is not what dying did to them that we remember, but what they have done to our thoughts on death. Like this girl they showed how the spirit, so much stronger than the body, was not only independent of their physical deterioration, but made of it the means of growth and even of happiness. They showed that there was something in the ending of their life that made the whole of all that went before deeper and more full of meaning, and assured us of its fulfilment in another phase of existence.

Poets have spoken of the 'lightening before death' and all those who remain with the dying have seen this, sometimes minutes, sometimes hours before the actual moment of death. Recently the Matron of the Hospice in which we work was sitting beside a devout old man and was able to watch in quietness something that those who are busy or blind with grief must often miss – a moment of quietness just before he died, when all the lines on his face gradually faded, leaving an expression of immense happiness and peace. As she described it I found myself thinking that what she saw was exactly the same expression of peace that comes when a loved one arrives after anxious waiting, perhaps never better expressed than in China in the twelfth century BC:

> I climbed the hill just as the new moon showed,
> I saw him coming on the southern road.
> My heart lays down its load.

I remember someone who suddenly, just before he lost consciousness, looked up and smiled with a look of gaiety that made me say ruefully to myself afterwards, 'But he looked amused!' It was as if he had said to me 'Why did we make such a fuss? Everything is all right after all.' Only much later did I really find the same for myself.

When we see the dying look like this we know that they are moving into a new dimension where time no longer moves inexorably to parting but rather encloses in safety the procession of moments in which we all trip and stumble, never able to catch our joys as they fly. These moments together still exist in this dimension beyond, along with all their effects upon our work and life. It seems to me that it is the very intensity of the moments of parting, the weakness and weariness of the end of a long illness and of the problems endured together, that give these moments their depth and power. We see people go through a lifetime of experience in a few weeks, a long time is fulfilled in a short time. They seem to know a timeless 'Now' when all the moments of time are held in stillness.

As all the decisions and acts that have brought us to this present moment are summed up in our smallest act, so all we have loved are there too, inextricably bound up in all that we are. We bring them with us just as they take us with them. But we can choose how we bring them, whether it shall be in resentment or in re-conciliation. We can look back and tell the story of our past as a series of failures or we can find in it instead a series of rewards and joys. So with our memories of our dead, the emphasis we place can give us fresh wounds or change them into blessings, can weigh down our daily living with regret or lift it with gratitude.

I am saying all this not only as a doctor and as someone who remembers many friends but also from my own religious conviction. When one of my friends was dying and grieving that parting could only hurt those he loved, he suddenly looked up at the crucifix on the wall of the ward . . . 'I can see my Saviour. . . .' For the Christian the cross is the centre of all centres, the place where time and eternity meet and all our griefs and failures are transformed. It teaches that we can indeed see God in every grief and in every pain, and in seeing this, see beyond to the victory over them won for us all. Other faiths see this differently, but we can all meet as we find in grief not only that we belong with all other men but that we belong with God also. We and those we love, wherever we may be, are safe.

10 Clinical Theology: a Survey

Hugh Melinsky

Hugh Melinsky is the Honorary Editor of the Institute of Religion and Medicine, having been a member from its inception. From 1961 to 1968 he served as part-time Chaplain to the Norfolk and Norwich Hospital, and he still maintains some links with the chaplaincy service. He was for four years Director of the Norwich Branch of the Samaritans. He is now Canon Missioner in charge of lay training in the Norwich diocese.

The background of this chapter is a consultation which was held in Durham in January 1969 organized by the Rev. G. C. Harding and attended by Dr Brian Lake and other founder-members of the Clinical Theology movement. Any views, however, expressed in this chapter are entirely the responsibility of the author.

'Clinical Theology' is a name associated with a movement of clinical pastoral care founded and directed by Dr Frank Lake. Dr Lake served as a medical missionary in India from 1937, specializing in tropical parasitology. From 1940 to 1950 he became involved in the psychological testing first of army officers and then of medical students. As Superintendent of the Christian Medical College at Vellore in South India he assisted Dr Florence Nichols to establish a psychiatric unit there, and in the process made his first contact with dynamic psychiatry. The Church Missionary Society suggested that he specialize in the field of psychiatry, and so he studied for a Diploma in Psychological Medicine at the University of Leeds.

In 1958, with a centre established at Nottingham, there began a series of seminars which in the subsequent ten years have included well over 5,000 people, both clergy and laity. Originally only clergy attended, but in recent years there have been as many lay people as clergy and ministers. The programme laid down one three-hour seminar every three weeks over a period of two years. The movement expanded as members who had successfully negotiated this course acted in turn as tutors in their own localities, sometimes providing courses a good deal shorter than the original. Much of Dr Lake's teaching material is to be found in his own *magnum opus* of 1,200 pages published in 1966 under the title *Clinical Theology*.[1]

The purpose of the seminars was to help clergy fulfil their pastoral duties more effectively in caring for people who came to them with affliction of mind and spirit. Most of the severely mentally ill do not find their way to clergymen in the first place because their illness is spotted and they are led towards proper hospital treatment. A large number of troubled people do, however, present to their ministers mild depressions and anxieties and symptoms of neurosis and stress, sometimes expressed in spiritual terms. The other main group of people who seek help from clergy are those for whom the psychiatrist can do no more, or those who the psychiatrist says are not for him. According to Dr Lake, about a third of all those who have received psychiatric treatment still need supportive help afterwards; and, since it is reckoned that something like one in eight of the population suffers illness which is of the mind/spirit rather than of the body, there cannot possibly be enough professional psychiatric and psychotherapeutic help available. Thus much will fall inevitably on clergy who care for the deep things of their people's personalities.

It soon became apparent in the early seminars that the students were not concerned primarily with their parishioners' problems; they were really troubled about their own, some so severely as to be themselves in risk of breakdown. Thus the groups were not just classes for intellectual learning; they became groups in which many of the dynamics of mental illness and spiritual affliction were experienced in the relationships of the members. The major achievement of the movement has been the insight it has imparted to its students about their own personality problems and their religious interpretation – an insight which is vital before much can be done in helping others with theirs.

Up to 1950 the clergy had been given little to help them at their theological colleges. Some colleges had a few formal lectures from a psychiatrist, but staffs generally treated such matters with a distant respect, if not a lofty disdain. As a result many clergy treated troubled people with textbook answers about sin, and if they allowed the troubles to enter their own lives more deeply, found themselves in difficulty about handling the powerful feelings which these troubles engendered.

This anxiety on the part of the clergy was a principal reason for the initial success of Clinical Theology. Many of them were aware of the compulsive aspects of human behaviour which did not cease with conversion in the case of their parishioners or with ordination in their own case. A homosexual parishioner still had his homosexuality to contend with, and if a clergyman was to help him at any deep level it was possible that the pastoral process would uncover homosexual traits in the helper. How could the helper be helped? Clinical Theology offered an answer.

The movement, from its early days, ran into heavy criticism. Its very title was disliked by some theologians as presuming to offer *the only* system of pastoral care, whereas both its theology and its psychology were drawn from selected portions of those very large fields. For theological guidance Dr Lake looks principally to Job, St John's gospel, St Paul's epistle to the Romans, St John of the Cross, Kierkegaard, Simone Weil and Martin Buber. His psychological mentors are Freud and the neo-Freudians, Klein, Fairbairn, Sullivan and Guntrip. Since there are great divergences amongst theologians and psychiatrists in their own fields, it is hardly to be expected that any one mortal could lead these two contentious disciplines to a happy marriage. The period of courtship looks like being a long one.

A good deal of criticism came from psychiatrists, not least from Christian psychiatrists, partly because the psychiatric background was so selective; partly because Dr Lake, particularly in his published diagrams, seemed to make a definitive mapping of the human personality; and partly because Dr Lake made connexions and equations between the two disciplines which seemed to many people to be premature and superficial. These matters call for further consideration.

Some of the founder-members of the movement now admit that in the early days they did not pay enough attention to psychiatrists and sociologists. They found it hard to gain a hearing from them. They admit also that the movement expanded too fast without enough proper supervision. Psychiatrists are very sensitive to members of other helping professions who appear to be trespassing on their professional preserves, and do not seem to be impressed by the analogy of 'psychiatric first-aid' to be administered by trained volunteers in the same way as a Red Cross worker can staunch a wound or splint a fractured limb or administer the kiss of life to a drowning person.

Psychiatrists may answer that first-aid work does not require the theory set out in Dr Lake's massive book, and some of his colleagues admit that in the early years there was too great an emphasis on the intellectual approach. Nevertheless the task remains of bridging the gulf between the two disciplines, or rather, of interpreting the insights of the one to the other. Psychiatry and religion both claim to be actively concerned with the deep ills of human nature, and people who are so afflicted will very often seek help both from ministers of religion and from medical practitioners. In the interest of those who suffer it is necessary that both kinds of practitioners talk to each other with a view to understanding each other's approach and the resources which each can offer.

It is fairly easy to find fault with Dr Lake's system of Clinical Theology both in theory and in practice, but any critic does well to remember that he was a pioneer; that like most pioneers he was under constant attack from established authorities (in this case from church and medicine alike); that his sharpest critics had nothing better to offer; and that his system obviously answered a real need felt by clergy and laity who wanted to do their pastoral job better and found that this meant that before they could deal with other people's problems they had to have a close look at their own first. Any criticism advanced in these pages is done so in full awareness of these factors.

The theological aspect

Dr Lake expresses in his book a healthy dislike for theological systems (even if he is more partial to psychological ones). He takes his stand on the orthodox doctrine of God the Holy Trinity whose 'family life' is the ground of all our human relationships, internal and external. He takes a poor view of (and attaches a schizoid label to) Christian thinkers who would reduce God to an impersonal ground of being. In fact he defines pastoral care as 'an inter-personal relationship in the name of a personal God'.

Dr Lake describes how, while at Vellore, he was searching for a model of the normal dynamic circle of personal relationships and asked Emil Brunner, the Swiss theologian, who was visiting the Medical College, for guidance. Brunner directed him to a study of the person of Christ as portrayed in St John's gospel. Thus the 'norm' of human nature is to be sought in terms of a reciprocal relationship of love between Father and Son mediated by the Holy

Spirit. The work of Christ as the Son is the dynamic outflow of personal being and well-being consequent on this relationship. We may say that Jesus Christ was the only truly 'normal' person.

As might be expected of a doctor who worked for the Church Missionary Society, the crucifixion and resurrection of Christ are central to his theology and also to his concept of pastoral care. He agrees with Thurneysen's assertion that 'All true pastoral care is concerned with proclaiming the forgiveness of sin' but the redemptive effects of the cross must not be limited to sinners only; reconciliation is also for all sufferers. Past hurt, deeply repressed, which causes the sufferer to condemn faith as a delusion – this also is confronted by the fact of Christ's cross.

Dr Lake insists that the faith by which Christians lay hold of the re-relating which Christ has achieved for us and in spite of us – that this faith must be a living and dynamic thing, and that it must inevitably remove any superiority in the pastor's attitude. Being wide-awake to the dangers of sectarian religiosity, he underlines the danger, not unknown in evangelical circles, of erecting the doctrine of 'justification by faith' into a saving work, when salvation becomes limited to those who feel themselves able to subscribe to a particular interpretation of a biblical doctrine.[2]

He is equally severe in his criticism of certain aspects of the Catholic tradition of confession and pastoral counselling (both Roman and Anglican), when, for example, the technique of the confessional does not allow time for a lengthy listening to the life background of the penitent. It is important to distinguish between rational guilt which can be confessed and absolved, and irrational fantasies which well up from deeply repressed mental pain, and only time and patience in listening to the penitent's life story will provide enough means for the distinction.[3]

It follows that baptism is the assurance of a man's right standing and belonging, his being in Christ, and that this assurance is the basic answer to every human anxiety and insecurity. The task of the church is to make this fact of belonging real and ever-present, and of the Christian healer to make it present despite overwhelming waves of mental pain. There is no simple and certain cure for some forms of affliction. The Christian 'cure' is for the sufferer to come to terms with his affliction in the light of the cross of Christ. Of this, the waters of baptism are a powerful symbol.

The principal means of Christian therapy is friendship, a quality, indeed the only quality, which makes life worth living for those who have decided otherwise. This is a task not only for the professional Christian therapist but also for the whole Christian congregation.

The psychological aspect

Neurotic anxiety, of the sort that clergymen or compassionate lay-people like Samaritan volunteers are likely to meet is, for Dr Lake, the echo of the pain of long-lost relationships, and in particular the warm, caring, affection of a mother for her infant child. In this basic assumption Dr Lake follows the findings of Melanie Klein and Ronald Fairbairn, maintaining that a child's first quest is for a person rather than for the sexual gratification of classical Freudianism.

Clinical Theology is not much concerned for the severer psychoses, nor for the therapy of drugs or electric shock. This at once puts it out of court for many psychiatrists who see by far the greatest part of mental illness as being curable, within the next ten years, by chemo-therapy. This is not the occasion to raise the crucial question of 'drugs or dynamics'. Such a distinction is probably a misleading one in any case. As an American doctor wrote of the psychosomatic approach to illness:

> To me it seems to be a *meaningless* question to ask whether the physiological process is causing the psychological state, or the psychological state is causing the physiological process. Both are arbitrary descriptions, in arbitrary terms, of a particular global process, and it is for this reason that I think long discussions about what is most important or basic in such a process are irrelevant, misleading, and quixotic.[4]

The fact remains that many ex-patients still seek the supportive help of suitable clergymen and lay-people; that many people bear a great amount of affliction whom the psychiatrists say they cannot help and for whom they prescribe tranquillizing drugs; and that anyhow there is not enough professional psychotherapeutic help available in this country to give the time necessary for the sort of personal care with which Dr Lake is concerned.

His three principal categories of illness (or affliction, as he prefers to call it) are:

(1) the hystero-schizoid pattern, deriving from a fear of death and non-being;

(2) the paranoid pattern, deriving from a profound sense of meaninglessness; and

(3) the depressive pattern, deriving from a deep sense of guilt and condemnation.

He treats the schizoid pattern at greatest length, but begins with the depressive, and so we shall follow his order.

But first, reference must be made to lysergic acid (LSD 25) because this plays a major part in Dr Lake's argument. From the beginning of his psychiatric practice, some three years before the start of the Clinical Theology movement, he used this drug clinically to enable his patient to uncover primitive infantile emotions, particularly those of pain and deprivation. The latter part of the interview is devoted to the patient's relating, with the friendly support of the psychiatrist, these primitive experiences to subsequent painful situations.

A great deal hangs on this interpretation, and Dr Lake is convinced that LSD can uncover clear memories going back to the journey of a baby through the birth-passages of its mother. He produces some striking evidence of patients' recollections under LSD being confirmed from their mothers' own memories hitherto untold. Doubts have been cast on the value of this kind of recollection, even as to whether an infant's brain is neurologically capable of storing and reproducing such impressions. In any case Dr Lake seems bold in the way in which he accepts this kind of testimony almost verbatim. Such a hot-line to the heart of the unconscious seems too good to be true.

The reactive depression, he claims, can be helped by the 'clinical theologian'. Indeed, the dividing line between the endogenous and the reactive depression is far from clear. Depression stems basically from an infantile rage resulting from a sense of rejection and frustration turning in on itself, though there may also be hereditary and biochemical factors involved. The help which the theologian can give (based on the invariable ministry of listening) finds its pattern in the psalmist, who pours out his soul, freely admitting his heaviness of spirit; who takes God to task for his depression; who continues to affirm that this is God's world; who clings to one outside himself; and counsels patience – an active passivity.[5] The depressed person is not humble but proud, clinging to a selfish hate. Relief consists in diminishing his neurotic guilt; establishing his actual sin; and helping him find true forgiveness, and a new affection.

Dr Lake has no hesitation in forging firm links between depression and 'accidie', the medieval name for sloth, one of the seven deadly sins. It was well known as a state of restlessness and an inability either to work or to pray. A whole chart is devoted to analysing the make-up of accidie from theologians across the centuries and the pattern is found to be essentially similar to the dynamics of depressive anxiety. Although there are many fascinating similarities, the field on both sides is so wide that many readers have complained that this equation is too easy; the factors have been selected to suit the equation; and terms must be carefully examined against their background before they can be exchanged across the frontier of their own discipline. There is substance to these criticisms.

Dr Lake's second main concern is with the 'hysteric' pattern of personality. He traces the cause back to an extreme pain of infant separation which in later life produces behaviour designed to gain and keep active acceptance at any cost – and the cost can be extremely high. There must be few parish priests who have not had to contend with a hysterical woman parishioner 'pretending to be what she is instead of being it'. Sexual relationships are often impaired by sexual fantasies. In severe cases the mental strain is converted into physical symptoms like blindness, paralysis, and loss of memory: the extreme state is that of the hysterical psychopath who shows no feeling for any of the standards of civilized behaviour. The hysteric is not much loved by psychiatrists, and hysteria is given little attention in the standard textbooks of psychiatry.

If hysteria is a cry against terrifying loneliness, the Christian gospel speaks of a God who is near and cares. How can this nearness be made a reality? There are no gimmicks by way of an answer. There is worship and prayer and meditation on the scriptures. There is also Christian friendship. The befriending of a hysteric is fraught with difficulty, and it must be both kind and stern. The pastor must limit the time allotted and must learn to say 'No' while it is still reasonable. He must introduce the person into some form of group activity, which in turn means giving the group some training in how to cope with demands and tantrums. Dr Lake suggests that trained helpers should act in pairs so that they can consult with each other; and he emphasizes the importance of supportive prayer-groups. The prognosis is never certain and often produces surprises.

Hysteria is only one form, for Dr Lake, of a more basic and more pervasive personality disorder which he calls 'schizoid' or 'split' (to be distinguished from the classical schizophrenic). The split originates in infancy in stress which passes the bounds of bearing, and this may be traced back as far as a birth with particularly difficult labour. It is always associated with the absence, or apparent absence, of a mother's warm affection, and is frequently found among offspring of coldly intellectual parents. The split, originating in a loss of person-centredness, spreads to involve other persons and things. There is a dramatic about-turn. Longing for life turns into longing for death; desire for pleasure turns into desire for pain; compulsive attachment to people turns into a revulsion from people. Life is filled with a sense of dread. The 'I' has lost its 'Thou'; the person feels depersonalized; life has no meaning or purpose; only apathy, weariness and a sense of tedious futility. The result is frequently anxiety over an inability to commit oneself to anything, especially to marriage, to work, or to religion.

This state of futile and meaningless existence has been extensively explored and described by the existentialist philosophers and writers whose patron saint is Søren Kierkegaard, though Dr Lake takes the line further back to Job and Pascal. Of such basic importance is this position that Dr Lake is prepared to say, 'It is at this ontological level of statement that psychiatry communicates with theology.'[6]

The psychiatrists want to abolish anxiety, claims Dr Lake, whereas the clinical counsellor wants to make its meaning clear. He quotes Simone Weil: 'The extreme greatness of Christianity lies in the fact that it does not seek a supernatural remedy for suffering but a supernatural use for it.' The first act of faith is resignation, because the schizoid sufferer is terrified to commit himself to anything, let alone faith. Faith is choosing to gaze Godwards in total darkness. Despair before God is the first act of faith and 'to find the absolute one must proceed, not from doubt, but from despair' (in Kierkegaard's memorable words).

In answer, Christianity proclaims a God who gives meaning, in and beyond despair; a Christ who has himself entered the depths of human affliction and dereliction; a baptism which is the death and burial of the old self; a Holy Communion which continues the dynamic union of all Christians with Christ; and the church which is, or ought to be, under its chief pastor, a healing fellowship. If the fear of dread is fear ultimately about the nature of God, it will not be easy for the healer to remain personally uninvolved.

The paranoid personality is basically similar, for Dr Lake, to the schizoid in that it is shaped in its earliest months by the unbearable loss of well-being. There are many graduations of the paranoid condition, from the parson with a load of chips on his shoulder, to the patient in hospital claiming to be God. (Dr Lake mentions that once he had two patients in adjacent beds each claiming to be God.) Unlike the schizoid state there is no sense of loss of being, though there is a devastating loss of a sense of well-being. The paranoid patient or parishioner, having buried the extreme persecutory pain deep in his unconscious, reconstructs the world on a delusional basis so that everything becomes threatening, mysterious, and elusive. All characters are suspicious and all acts hostile.

Such people are notoriously hard to help, because although they ask for help they will resent it. To accept that the therapist has the ability to effect a cure is itself a threat to the patient's own delusion of superiority. The redemptive task is to accept the person as he is, delusions and all. It is hopeless to tackle the delusions on a rational basis, but pastoral care may in time help the sufferer to understand something of what has called the delusions into being. Dr Lake sees the Christian as having additional resources to help in this task. A trained psychotherapist has to bear a tremendous burden of mistrust and suspicion directed at him by the patient, and in the end has only his own personal resources to stand it. The Christian pastor, however, has more. He proceeds from a 'holy insecurity'; he has learned that being persecuted is an important element in blessedness; and he is open to inspiration from outside himself.

The ecclesiastical aspect

It should be clear by now that Dr Lake holds a high doctrine of the church. Its fellowship, its trained pastors, its sacraments, scriptures and spiritual discipline are all elements in the pastoral care and cure of the mentally and spiritually afflicted. He is critical of the normal congregation for not accepting troubled people as they really are but only under a guise of respectable middle-class normality. He insists that the church should go out in the wilderness to meet the solitary wanderer. Drawing on his experience of small therapeutic groups he urges church leaders to set an example by themselves conducting small groups of clergy and laity who have encountered some major emotional crisis which is hindering their daily living – and quotes the words from the consecration service of bishops in the Church of England; 'Hold up the weak, heal the sick, bind up the broken, bring again the outcasts, seek the lost.'

Training for this kind of pastoral care is best given through the experience of 'group dynamics'. This, briefly described, is an exercise in which about ten people undertake, for a period of days, simply to be a member of the group and to observe the behaviour of the group. After a couple of days the veneer of politeness wears thin and some of the deep motivating forces of group behaviour become all too visible. Real insight can be gained about the way these forces actually operate in and between individuals in a group, and also between groups, and deep involvement in the situation gives opportunity for an opening up and development of the personality.

This kind of training group has been found to be of great value for those who undertake the befriending of disturbed and distressed people. The experience of the Samaritans is that befriending severely depressed or dispirited clients makes heavy demands on volunteers and is likely to show up the weak points in a helper's personality; but that these sensitive points can best be helped in a small group where the truth can be spoken in love.

In more specifically ecclesiastical ways Dr Lake has found membership of a prayer group a valuable aid for the hysteric; and neurotically obsessive people have been helped by the sheer givenness of the Holy Communion, of Bible meditation, and of the laying-on of hands. Above all, time is necessary for listening, and Dr Lake attaches considerable importance to the keeping of a full and orderly record of a patient's history.

Problems raised

This bald summary of Dr Lake's position hardly does justice to the richness of material which he has gathered into the 1,200 pages of his book. He is frequently moved to long excursuses taking the form of a meditation on the Bible or on some spiritual writer, or even a sermon. There are many flashes of insight sparked off by high-tension contact between the fields of theology and psychiatry. But there are also links made between the two disciplines which are too simple. To claim that justification by faith is the remedy for depression[7] is a dangerously misleading sort of shorthand which is calculated to enrage both theologian and psychiatrist. It is true that Dr Lake explicates at length what he means by both terms, but they are drawn from different disciplines which attempt to describe different aspects of human experience, and use different categories of language on different logical levels, and they do not take kindly to such a shot-gun marriage.

To identify accidie with depression is to beg as many questions as it answers.[8] It is certainly possible to draw out an illuminating list or chart of similarities, but 'depression' is a wide field, and the charge can easily be laid of selecting those features which match up with the corresponding theological factors.

To identify Mary Magdalene as a hysteric because at the end she wishes to cling to the Master[9] is to go some way beyond the evidence; so also with the Syro-Phoenician woman as 'hysterical in her need and clinging; afflicted and ready to shrink away like a beaten cur into a cringing schizoid detachment';[10] so also is identifying the hypocrisy of the Pharisees with a generous use of dissociative personality mechanisms.[11]

Dr Lake has little doubt about the actuality of the 'death-wish' (although he admits that Freud only postulated it as a hypothesis), and identifies its origin in an experience of unbearable pain at birth.[12] He goes on to interpret the 6th, 7th and 8th chapters of the Epistle to the Romans as describing how the death of Christ 'is the overcoming in God-made-man, of the ultimate terrors of death of the spirit': it is, in fact, the killing of the death-wish. Again, this kind of equation is likely to satisfy as few psychiatrists as it will theologians. A distinguished psychiatrist recently described the death-wish as heady stuff and warned philosophers against playing with it ingeniously, undeterred by its meaninglessness.[13] Theologians also would maintain that being made conformable to the death of Christ, even if it could be taken to mean 'a death in us, both to our hysterical fear of death, and to our schizoid love of it'[14] means a great deal else besides.

Dr Lake also draws attention to a close correspondence between the 'dark night of the soul', classically described by St John of the Cross, and the schizoid sufferer detaching himself from visible symbols of security, and so experiencing an intensification of separation-anxiety.[15] But St John's writings are set in a particular context. They are by a contemplative for others who would follow the mystical way. The final goal is clear, which is union with God; self-denial is not of sins or pleasures but of perfectly normal things, spiritual as well as material (the dark night of sense); the renunciation of these may lead to a hearing of voices or seeing of visions, but then a period of terrible spiritual troubles must be endured (the dark night of soul), and a very few who survive will be privileged to experience 'union' or 'transformation' or even 'deification'. St John is well known for his keen psychological insight, but the context of his work is a spiritual tradition very different, one would suppose, from that of most of Dr Lake's patients.

Dr Lake is happy to describe St John of the Cross as an existential writer. This is a mark of high praise because Clinical Theology is nurtured very much on existentialist thinking. Pascal, Kierkegaard, Simone Weil, R. D. Laing are principal figures, and it is in connexion with the last-named that Dr Lake nails his colours to the existentialist mast: 'It is at this ontological level of statement that psychiatry communicates with theology, or at least would do so if theologians were prepared to listen and search for answers.'[16] It is impossible to examine this claim fully or fairly in a few sentences. In any case the name 'existentialism' applies to a broad movement of thought from the deeply religious Kierkegaard to the atheistic Sartre. Suffice it to say here that the movement is a pessimistic one, typical of the dark side of the twentieth century and the disillusionment of two world wars. Both Kierkegaard and Simone Weil, for all their religious insights, were deeply neurotic characters, the former finding the genesis of religion in despair, and the latter dying at the age of thirty-four as a result of a self-denial which almost amounted to a prolonged act of suicide. There is, therefore, a built-in compatibility between this approach to theology and the psychological approach to human affliction.

Conclusion.   Issues raised

Clinical Theology is a pioneer movement in the church, and seems now to have reached the end of its first phase. It has been heavily criticized, and as a system it is open to criticism. (What system is not?) Nevertheless it has made a signal contribution to the life of the church, not least by clearly sign-posting some of the pit-falls in a hitherto little-explored no-man's-land. So by way of conclusion we may point to five lessons to be learned from a survey of the ten years of this movement.

Academically speaking, it has been a brave attempt to marry the diverse disciplines of theology and psychology, but it has tried to do this over too selective an area and on too uniform a level. Indeed it may not even be possible to work out a 'system' which can do justice to both disciplines (remembering especially Dr Lake's dislike of systems). It may be necessary, for some time to come, to be content with an interchange of insights between the two disciplines which can illuminate, each in its own way, dark corners of the human situation. Further, it may be necessary to pay more attention to the sociological sciences as well. Other pages in the present volume criticize the one-to-one dimension of psychotherapeutic care. A parish priest who is reduced to a near-breakdown because his village has been condemned to economic death needs to have his problem considered in the light of social as well as psychological factors. A far greater interchange of thought and experience needs to take place between these disciplines at every stage of professional training.

Clinical theology has cast much light on the manner of learning. The deep things of the human personality are not open to inspection, handling, and change like experiments in a laboratory or facts in a classroom. The pastor, counsellor, or psychotherapist is inevitably personally involved to some extent, and the wholeness of his parishioner or patient will depend accordingly on his own degree of wholeness. This cannot be learned: it can only be developed by experiential training. The theory underlying group-dynamics is of considerable importance. Is this a particular mode of operation of the Holy Spirit? Is the small supportive psychotherapeutic group in effect a prayer group? These questions call for further investigation, though not here.

What, indeed, *is* pastoral counselling? Is it a priestly function or is it a misleading myth? How is it related to the joyful proclamation of good news? Ought it not anyway to be set in the context of a Christian congregation with its on-going worship and fellowship? These are issues raised. The answers are not yet clear.

One practical issue is clear, namely the need for some 'resource-point' or 'resource-person' in the community. He (or they) would be known as someone to whom a person in trouble can go; he would be able to diagnose the nature of the trouble and refer the person to the best source of help available. The resource-point would also be a place where members from various helping professions could regularly meet for conversation across the frontiers. To some extent this is already taking place with meetings, for example, of doctors and clergy, or luncheon-clubs for clergy and social workers. The point would exist not only to help the community but also to help those who were helping the community. The nature of such a resource-point would depend very much on the local situation. No blue-print is possible.

A broader issue which emerges clearly from this survey is the need for some sort of standing organization to review methods and procedures. This would be able to examine the academic credentials of an organization and advise on the co-ordination of its work with other bodies concerned. It could save a great deal of frustration and overlapping effort.

Behind all these particular issues lies the question to which the Uppsala Conference found itself being driven: What is man? Both philosophical and theological thought wait on an answer to this question, some agreed map of what constitutes a human person and how he works, and fails to work. The World Council of Churches has appointed a working party under Canon David Jenkins to consider this crucial question, and the outcome of their investigations will be awaited with more than usual expectancy.

NOTES

1. Frank Lake, *Clinical Theology*, Darton, Longman and Todd 1966
2. *C.T.*, p. 77
3. *C.T.*, p. 236
4. *Psychophysiological Aspects of Cancer*, ed. E. M. Weyer, New York Academy of Sciences 1966, p. 1053
5. E.g. Psalm 42
6. *C.T.*, p. 601
7. *C.T.*, p. 107
8. *C.T.*, p. 111
9. *C.T.*, p. 450
10. *C.T.*, p. 826
11. *C.T.*, p. 461
12. *C.T.*, p. 792
13. Charles Rycroft in *New Society*, 25 September 1969, p. 488
14. *C.T.*, p. 792
15. *C.T.*, p. 842

11 With Love to the USA

R. A. Lambourne

Dr Robert Lambourne served during the war as a Regimental Medical Officer, following this with nine years in general practice in Birmingham, his home town. In 1956 he began deeper study in the philosophy and theology of healing at Birmingham University, gaining the degree of Bachelor of Divinity by thesis. In 1962 he left general practice for the full-time study of psychological medicine. He was instrumental in the formation of the Department of Pastoral Studies at Birmingham University, and now lectures in its postgraduate Diploma course which brings together the disciplines of theology, psychology, and sociology.

The following chapter first appeared in the USA as an article in the *Journal of Religion and Health*, and is reproduced here by kind permission.

My interest is in medico-theological matters. The purpose of this article is to report my reactions following a three weeks' visit to the United States in which a few selected experiences at certain centres supplemented many years' reading of American literature on practical training for the ministry and especially clinical pastoral care and pastoral psychology. It must be admitted that this reading had prejudiced me. I had for years envied the sophistication, imagination, and expenditure of resources by the American churches in the area of clinical pastoral training and counselling. On the other hand, I had come to be exasperated by the almost total lack of theological thrust displayed in their so-called dialogue with psychoanalysis. The disparity between the flood of literature on pastoral psychology and the trickle of writing on the theology of pastoral care during the last twenty years has been only too obvious. It seemed that theologians could find no middle way between hostility and obsequiousness to the therapists, and that as a consequence systematic theologians rarely contributed to the debate in any vigorous fashion.

For this and other reasons which will be mentioned later, it seemed to me that what was emerging was a virulent psychological pietism which, despite the fact that it was training hospital chaplains and using them in training, characteristically never said anything radical about the central concepts and structures of medicine. It looked from the literature as if the claimed dialogue with medicine had not yet begun, and that the much hailed dialogue with psychiatry was only a psychiatric monologue. Worse still, it looked as if this so-called dialogue had resulted in a collusion between theology and psychotherapy which was partly maintained by a neglect of, and even hostility towards, organically-minded medicine. Thereby the building of a sound bridge between theology and medicine was being deferred by those very persons who might at first sight have been thought to be most likely to finish it. This, then, was my impression from reading the literature.

My visit suggested that, while there are many in the USA who are aware of these difficulties, and while there are many exciting experiments in concepts, practical pastoralia and practical pastoral training, which together might answer all my criticisms, it still remains true that the main effort in the theory, teaching, and practice of pastoral care and in medico-theological dialogue is very unsatisfactory. This is not because of any lack of competent men or competent teaching techniques, but because of conceptual deficiencies which stem in their turn from the absence of tough dialogue between medicine and theology, and from the much overprotected situation of the analysts, counsellors and pastoral experts who had been the teaching pastors' mentors. What is meant by this will be explained below.

There seems to be a split, perhaps a growing split, between those who are teaching practical theology through pastoral counselling and clinical pastoral care (Group A) and those who are teaching it through field work in depressed urban situations (Group B). The former lean heavily, and sometimes exclusively, on psychology. The latter lean heavily, and sometimes exclusively, on sociology. The former teach sensitivity by psychological interpretation in controlled unstructured groups, the latter by selected exposure to cultural shock. The danger seems to be that, because of some grave deficiencies in the theory and practice of the former group, the latter will react from its quietism to a political activism which is sociologically informed but personally insensitive. The fact that the former is taught predominantly in an academic or hospital setting while the latter is taught predominantly outside these situations, and often by a different group of teachers, makes for the dangerous possibility of this split remaining unhealed. This would mean an impoverishment for both.

So far as the medico-theological dialogue is concerned there is, however, a third group (Group C) of thelogians who, noting that the unparalleled American sophistication in training for hospital chaplaincy work has been so entangled in counselling that it has rarely if ever said anything prophetic about the medical structures within which it counselled, has turned aside and interested itself in the concepts underlying medicine and medical education and in the philosophical and theological problems thrown up by modern medicine in the sphere of medical ethics. Unfortunately, this group is scarcely affecting the mainstream of clinicopastoral education which is largely in the hands of Group A. In the long run, Group C's concern for being a serving Christian presence in the centre of medicine may mean the development of a theology of healing which takes matter as seriously as it does persons. They may thus remedy some of the defects in the present theology of pastoral care, which operates almost entirely with a psychic-affective type of christology, doing scant justice to either Christ's incarnation or to logos christology, about which more will be said later.

There are, then, three groups with dangerous gaps between them. Group A concentrates on self-development at the expense of a neglect of justice and the creative stewardship of matter. Group B concentrates on justice at the expense of a neglect of self-development and the creative stewardship of matter. Group C, in its effort to engage medicine in a tough dialogue, might, if it can overcome its understandable prejudice against the others, provide the necessary bridges between all three, for medicine is obviously concerned with the first and the third, and under the pressure of social rights is increasingly having to take note of social justice and thus of the interests of the second group.

If we now turn our attention to the first of these groups (Group A), that which is concerned with clinical pastoral care and pastoral counselling, it seems that it is the most powerful of the three in theological education and yet may be having the most difficulties in revising its concepts and practices. For these are well entrenched in departments of seminaries and divinity schools, in a mass of literature, in buildings, funds, professorial titles and appointments, and a highly self-selected network of interdisciplinary personal relationships reflecting much previous creative experience. The other two groups are comparatively young and weak, work in less protected environments, and perhaps for these very reasons may have to be more realistic and thus more adaptable. The question is, what sharp conceptual and practical changes may be required if Group A, with its rich talents and resources, is to make as valuable a contribution in the future as it has in the past?

The first necessity is for all concerned to recognize the extent to which the dialogue between theology and psychotherapy has been a tribalistic one which has concealed implicit value judgments, value judgments which, if they had been taken really seriously, would have raised the problems of justice which now exercises Group B particularly. The reason for this excessive tribalism lies in the special conditions in which psychoanalysis and counselling skills were developed. These conditions, of which the Jewish professional community of the late nineteenth century and the academics of the mid-western American campus between the wars provide good examples, provided a maximum of openness between the two or more participants within a highly enclosed situation. It may well have been Gentile discrimination which forced Freud and his followers to find an outlet for their creative genius which did not require the political and economic involvement which was denied them. Certainly the consulting-room situation, which always has an artificial flavour, was developed in psychoanalysis to provide a ghetto situation by the determined policy of the analyst in going out of his way not to meet the worldly contacts of the analysee, let alone exchange understandings with them of the patient's situation. Thus the undoubted gains of early psychoanalytical researchers were won in a situation which too easily tempted their successors to overlook the possibility that their claimed unconditional acceptance and love of the patient was operating in one of the most highly conditioned situations imaginable.

Thus began the separation of the theory and the art of loving from the theory and art of justice. Those who practised psychotherapy and those who learned from them did so in an artificial situation which protected them from the stings of cultural relativity, poverty, stupidity, unemployment, poor housing, and physical coercion. The marks of this are clearly visible after fifty years in the latest writings on the theology of pastoral care, despite the fact that existentialism and reality therapy have in the meantime substantially modified psychotherapeutic theory. In brief, these theologies of pastoral care have no place for justice except as a secondary phenomenon which follows man's non-acceptance of acceptance. This will be referred to again. The followers of Freud then took on unthinkingly a ghetto situation which was no chosen part of his life.

The Rogerian school of non-directive counselling, which was to rival Freud's influence in clinico-pastoral training and pastoral counselling, exhibits the same ghetto situation in which a highly intelligent, privileged, and relatively affluent group developed a theory and practice of counselling in an isolated situation where problems of cultural relativity, stupidity, poverty, physical coercion, and so on could be ignored, and thus encourage the participants to foster the delusion that they were engaged in a universal process to which problems of justice and power were either secondary or even irrelevant. Once again the theory and art of loving and acceptance were separated from the theory and art of justice and judgment. No wonder that both psychoanalysis and non-directive counselling could be used later to construct a particularly virulent form of secular pietism. No wonder that there is now the rift between Groups A and B mentioned above, for it would have been just such a strong sense of the ambiguity, in terms of ethics and justice, of every psychotherapeutic moment which could have provided the bridge between these two groups. The lack of this sense of being under judgment in the mainstream of psychoanalytic and Rogerian thought was later to prove a stumbling block when theologians made a determined attempt at a theological dialogue with these arts. The recent work of T. Oden and D. Browning shows this particularly well and will shortly be discussed.

There will be protests that the above description of the clinical pastoral and pastoral counselling movement in America does not do justice to the recent modifications produced by existential and reality therapy schools. These schools rightly insist that both therapist and patient must be vulnerable not only to each other, but also to each other in less artificial and more day-to-day situations. These protests may be just, but the point is that these new schools have as yet insufficiently modified the theory and practice of the main body of pastoral counselling and hardly modified at all the *theology* of pastoral care. (Nor, sad to say, does the vision for these modifications in psychotherapy appear to have come from a recovery of theological nerve, though it is thirty years since Reinhold Niebuhr's *Moral Man and Immoral Society* was available to spur us to ask about justice and pastoral counselling. Though to be fair it might be argued that Niebuhr, by sometimes seeming to fail to hold together God's love and God's justice, may have given the pastoral counsellors the inch they needed to take a mile.)

Two examples can now be given of how some of the best of recent theology of pastoral care is being built on old models of counselling which do not take sufficiently seriously problems of justice contained in the ambiguities existing in every therapeutic moment.

Professor T. Oden's work in *Kerygma and Counseling* and in *Contemporary Theology and Psychotherapy*[1] represents a very welcome example of a new type of high-level theological dialogue with psychiatry. Many of his insights are most instructive and acceptable, but the fact remains that the main thrust of his argument comes from positing a relationship between the emphatic acceptance of the therapist and the kerygma (i.e. the proclamation of the gospel). For Professor Oden, kerygma validates the empathic acceptance of the therapist by proclaiming that it is rooted in the act of God in Christ. But why has he started and stopped here? Might not an average reading of the New Testament suggest that the kerygma not only validates the empathic acceptance of the therapist, but also pronounces it to be under judgment? Even more, does not the kerygma both validate and put under judgment the *confrontation* which is inherent in every therapeutic moment because every moment, even a moment of silence, is a taking of a position which is known to be ambiguous? Does not every psychological interpretation, whether explicit in words or only implicit in an 'ugh', create a new situation which stands in need of a new interpretation; just as every new form of justice creates a new form of injustice? To transpose more of Reinhold Niebuhr's terms, is not complete acceptance of the client an impossible possibility, and does not every act of acceptance come under judgment? If this sounds theological nonsense, perhaps we may speak in a more secular way and as an example ask how any patient or any therapist in psychotherapy copes with the sense of injustice called forth by the knowledge that they are spending many hours in treatment and personal self-development while there are many others in different parts of the same country, let alone the same world, who are dying for want of simple medical treatment? The trouble is that the psychoanalytical and non-directive counselling movements have developed askew. By allowing their untenable claims to be practising a scientific non-value-judgment type of discipline to justify their practising in highly artificial and privileged situations, they have excluded themselves from those very realities of human situations which would have shown their claims to be untenable. Theologians can speak prophetically to this situation only if they will show how the gospel not only validates but also confronts the psychotherapist's work. The kind of sharp shift in the theology of pastoral care which is essential requires that someone – and who could do it better than Professor Oden? – should write a book on the theme 'Psychotherapeutic Interpretations, Prophecy, Ethics, and Kerygma'. This would give an ethico-political bridge between Group A and Group B.

A second book, which again epitomizes both the strength and weaknesses of recent writing on the theology of pastoral care, is Professor D. Browning's *Atonement and Psychotherapy*.[2] This fine work is delightful because here is someone taking patristics seriously in an attempt at real dialogue with psychotherapy. But once again the value of the book is seriously diminished because the human situation which is taken as a paradigm of atonement is a Rogerian counselling one which takes scarcely any note of the tension between justice and love in human situations. Thus it is no surprise that the author easily resolves the problem set for Anselm by the intensity with which he (Anselm) experienced the problem of how to reconcile God's justice with his love. Dr Browning does it by supporting Irenaeus from experience of the counselling situation where he claims judgment is a secondary phenomenon arising solely from the client's inability to accept the unconditional acceptance of the therapist. Thereby Professor Browning separates love and justice both in God and man. Thereby the possibility of God's primary justice being part of the same act as his primary love, and thus of man's justice being part of the same act as his love, is overlooked. But to do this is to encourage theologically the secular pietism which is already the bane of the counselling movement. I am not, of course, meaning to imply that Professor Browning and Professor Oden do not care about poverty, etc.; I know the contrary to be true. But these major theological works, by separating love from justice in God, using Rogerian counselling analogies, do not supply the correction required by Group A.

To correct it would mean first recognizing the implicit interpretation, and thus confrontation, in each psychotherapeutic word (or silence) and then using this, according to the same excellent methodology used by Dr Browning, as an analogy of the atoning work of the Divine word. This might then involve a second look at Anselm in which some of his unfashionable ideas about God's wrath might be illuminated by this psychotherapeutic experience and given back to the twentieth century. Those who met Christ were challenged to experience reality. They experienced at once both love and judgment – necessarily so because the love included a longing for a particular future state for the beloved. 'The wrath of the Lamb' hints how this strong longing for the good of the beloved means a wrathful love. The relevance of existential and reality concepts in correcting older theories of psychotherapy to a more balanced theory of atonement will be apparent.

In this connection, the philosophical anthropology of Martin Buber should prove a most useful tool, for his understanding of the 'confirming' element in dialogue insists from the start that dialogue always involves taking a stand as part of complete acceptance. This provides an ethical bridge which can become a bridge of politics and justice between the schools A and B mentioned above. Buber's insistence on the distinctive positions of therapist and client, even though the therapist is also vulnerable, is similarly wholesome. Finally, his insistence that one can have an I-thou dialogue with matter provides the possibility of correcting the tendency of the personalism in the clinico-pastoral training movement to gain enthusiasm by a contemptuous attitude to medical staff who cure predominantly by physical methods.

Several times it has been hinted that psychotherapeutic concepts and practices have gone astray because they were developed too much in a ghetto situation which encouraged unconscious tribalism and neglect of problems of justice. Now we must look more closely at this, for if mistakes have been made, we wish to correct them and prevent their recurrence. How has the mistake happened?

All people, and those in medicine and theology are by no means an exception, develop an anthropology–theology (the words are hyphenated to indicate that all anthropology involves theology and all theology involves anthropology) which reflects in part their own experience of reality developed within the general experience of reality of the profession to which they belong. The range of these experiences is necessarily limited by human limitations. It is further limited by personal deficiencies, by structures necessary for a useful professionalism, and by the need to narrow the field in order to explore and research in depth and detail. However, a dangerous limitation arises when the theology–anthropology derived from such limited experience is preached and practised by powerful professions without either an awareness of the extent to which limited experience has led to a limited anthropology–theology or a search for what were the unrecognized conditions of this experience.

The trouble gets worse when the unrecognized limitation gives rise to a theory which leads to practice which as a matter of professional discipline excludes the correcting experience required. The analyst's calculated self-exclusion from dialogue with the analysee's closest friends and relatives, or from meeting the analysee in his home or place of work or even socially, is a good example. The deliberate elimination of subjective elements from most medical research is another. The teaching of pastoral counselling to theological students on the seminary campus by teachers who were taught there by teachers who had learned it from others similarly trained is a third example. The result of this third situation is successive generations of dealing with persons with mental and feeling problems out of the social context of such persons and out of the context of physical disorders of the body. Successive generations of medical students and medical teachers who have learned their medicine in the protected atmosphere of the hospital full of quiescent patients horizontal in bed is an even more striking example with even more dangerous implications.

It follows from the above that as a matter of principle the education of teachers and students must always plan for a considerable degree of vulnerability to experiences which can challenge accepted understandings of man and reveal unrecognized understandings. It is never sufficient to arrange for vulnerability within the classes of experience which are recognized as important. The continual concentration of vulnerability within one carefully controlled area of life year after year in the same person, and generation after generation in the same profession, must be seen as a professional death warrant. Medical, theological, and psychoanalytical history demonstrates this only too well. Theologically, this is to take seriously the fact that Christ's incarnation is an expression of his obedience to be taught, by self-exposure, what was in man and what it was to be a man. His perfection is shown in his perfect obedience in being sent incarnate and vulnerable to be taught by the Father through the Spirit in particular situations what was in Man. He was taught what it was to be God's son, and shown the details of his role as Redeemer, Servant, Prophet, etc. The incident with the Syro-Phoenician woman, with its hint of an identity crisis for Jesus requiring a sharp revision of his understanding of these roles, can serve as a paradigm. He could not know beforehand that he would meet her, nor what he needed to be taught; but his general obedience through coming to a fully incarnate dialogue with the personal, social, material, political world was the condition for unplanned and unplannable acts of particular obedience. It is important to note that this is quite distinct from the idea of taking a theology or psychology or a medical anthropology into every corner of life. It points rather to discovering these things through and in every corner of life. In terms of training seminarians, it does not mean that they are given agency placings in society merely to practise the insights gained through theological studies or sensitivity groups in the seminary. It means channelling the learning experience of trans-cultural shock outside the seminary into the seminary. The same goes, of course, for the medical school and the teaching hospital.

It may be argued that, since by definition we do not know the nature of the correcting experience, it is impossible to arrange for it and therefore impossible to build it into professional experience and professional training. The same might be said of scientific discovery also. But it is surely possible to question assumptions and particularly any assumption or practice which *a priori* looks as if it protects the participants from a range of experiences. What is questioned verbally can then be questioned by some experimental training or practice. Also the value of permitting radical diversities in training, and thus openness to a variety of experiences, will be apparent. So will the need to look closely at any ideas and structures which distance the professional healer or saver from the situation where the sickness or sin may arise.

Is it wise, for example, to build a psychiatric hospital miles outside the city it serves and employ full-time psychiatrists who spend most of their working hours in the hospital and live outside the city? Is it wise to build special seminaries in green campuses and to stimulate personal maturation and increased sensitivity through common experiences within the seminary together with perhaps one or more other carefully chosen institution, as for example a clinico-pastoral experience in a psychiatric hospital? The last example is chosen because it illustrates the danger of making a truly broadening and opening-up experience universal within the training of professionals without noting that the key experience is given in very limiting circumstances which require challenge by different experiences. A closer look at the now fashionable urban experiences organized for theological seminarians is similarly required. Finally, whilst systematic education always properly requires selection of experiences for the learner (and this is unavoidable), some of the chosen exposures should be chosen just because the nature of the resultant experiences is highly unpredictable. One cannot, of course, plan future examinations to test learning of students from unpredictable experiences, and so no teaching institution will tolerate too much of this, especially since, where the healing profession concerned is socially powerful and influential, society itself will be the more concerned to see that candidates are vigorously examined. For this last reason it could happen that medical education might become more stereotyped than theological as the power of medicine increases and that of the church declines.

Mention of medicine reminds us of the third group of theologians and pastors engaged in some kind of debate with medicine. Members of Group C are concerned with two areas which often intermingle. These are medical ethics and the sociology of medicine. Because sociology tends to interest itself in different concepts of healing, with their resultant differences of medical planning involving in their turn differing priorities, there tends to be more discussion of values in medicine within the framework of social medicine than was so in the half-century which preceded the growth of departments of social medicine in medical schools. This has combined with the explosion of interest in medical ethics set off by spare-parts surgery to produce a rapidly growing group of doctors and theologians concerned with these matters. This discussion tends to lead eventually to much more penetrating questioning of the whole philosophy and practice of medicine than was produced by the clinico-pastoral theologians. This is most welcome, but would be even more so if these two groups were less divided. However, perhaps even more important than this is a subdivision within Group C of doctors and theologians whose interest is concentrated less on the personal ethical and personal social problems thrown up by medicine than on the philosophy of the physical and biological sciences which support medicine – sciences, which occupy the medical students in their pre-clinical years and decisively shape their style of being a doctor. These are the theologians and doctors who are prepared to take seriously the role of matter in the healing, saving plan of God and the work of Christ.

Those in this last sub-group of Group C are desperately needed to correct the balance in the medico-theological dialogue, which up to now looked suspiciously like that of a group of ministers of religion and psychiatrists who shared a reaction formation against the existential fear that their personality and their salvation might be in the hands of matter. Their apparent dialogue between medicine and theology may have taken place at the price of delaying conversation between the more representative centre of medicine and theology. The Incarnation seems to be a common stumbling block for such conversationalists, who often seem to operate a dualism between organic and psychological theories of personality formation and mental illness which plays the part in their total thinking which the older natural–supernatural dualism played for their forebears. Some of them will, it is feared, suffer a severe belief-crisis if clinical schizophrenia is healed by a pill! It seems that there is a persistent difficulty in taking sufficiently seriously the fully personal Incarnation of the Christ who not only had a body but was a body. Hence the difficulties for many Christians as for psychiatrists of a holding a soteriology which takes man's bodiliness seriously without lapsing into fatalism. Clinical medicine has a better record in this respect.

The end result has been that the clinico-pastoral movement has tended to encourage and stimulate Christian psychiatrists by using soteriological and healing models which made it harder for surgeons, molecular biologists, biochemists, internalists, and other central members of the healing profession to participate in the medico-theological dialogue. Consequently these central persons have up till now scarcely contributed to the search for common or at least mutually compatible models of healing and salvation. However, there are signs of a change, and within Group C are those who, sharing a common theory of knowledge and a common philosophical anthropology, are attempting to build a philosophy of medicine which leaves room for a distinctive Christian position, a position which is not basically a denial of the bodiliness of man and of the saving work of the body-person who was the Christ. These last theologians can, if they will join with the other groups of theologians concerned with the theology of pastoral care and the theology of healing, provide a group which is balanced and which has a systematic philosophy and theology which is sensitive to and inspired by the particular experiences of all three groups: those who are working in counselling and psychotherapy, those working in social and political situations, and those who are teaching and practising clinical medicine in hospital and outside.

To conclude, I should like to dwell upon what seems to me to be the key theological idea which the systematic theologian can bring to the theology of healing today. It is the strand of teaching of the living incarnate Logos epitomized by the christology of Colossians I and developed in Irenaeus. Here lies the possibility of a theory of knowledge which has room for a distinctive Christian contribution so that the Christian theory of knowledge and the Christian soteriology point to one common act of 'doing the truth' in which Christians participate in the work of the incarnate personal Christ's obedience and willing response under the law of *agapé* to the changing world of matter and persons which confronted him – to the Syro-Phoenician woman, to the incarnate Logos. A vulnerability in which we confirm the world we accept – to use Buber's terms – is the key to such 'doing the truth'. Here is a key theological concept for a contemporary medicine which is being transformed by, and in the grip of, a rapidly advancing understanding in the basic sciences and an accelerating technological revolution. There is here the possibility of an approach which could bring together the three schools of thought in the theology of healing. The existentialists suggested an interpersonal growth of self-understanding between people through shared openness, vulnerability and empathy. Buber, with his emphasis on 'confirming', provided the possibility of putting this within an ethico-political framework. In addition, by his insistence that the same I-thou dialogue could take place between man and matter, he provided a bridge between psychic personalism and physical medicine. Process theology based upon Whitehead seems to give a historical dimension to these previous philosophies, so that we can see individuals and communities by their combined acts of knowing and saving, their 'doing the truth', as participating in structuring a world moving towards a goal. This philosophical anthropology seems to leave room for a distinctive Christian contribution by suggesting that both the openness of man and his communities to this dialogue with man and with matter, and the confirming of man and matter in the dialogue, must follow the law of *agapé* as revealed by Christ. Such a kind of openness is a *kenosis*, a self-emptying, in which Christians sacrifice within the sacrifice of Christ. Only thus can the combined act of knowing and saving, of doing the truth, be a true doing of the truth.

Within such a general theological framework the community of healers, whether within or without the hospital, might be able to see themselves as participating in one act in Christ, though some of them, like medical biochemists or statisticians, seem sometimes to be concerned only with the pure knowledge and manipulation of matter, while others like psychiatrists seem to be sometimes concerned only in a verbal dialogue which saves. Here is the possibility of a theological model which can point to the presence of Christ in various acts of the healing community, and thus by implication to his absence from others, without producing thereby false dualisms, as for example between love and justice, mind and matter, psychological sensitivity and surgical impersonalism. Some such theological model could thus bring together for fruitful discussion Groups A, B, and C to produce a theology and practice of pastoral care which would do justice to the problem and to the opportunities for service.

This, then, is a call for redirection of the considerable personal and material resources in departments of pastoral theology. Perhaps there is an imbalance of professional chairs in these departments under such titles as 'Religion and Psychiatry' or 'Personality and Religion' which has not done justice to the pastoral ministry conceived of as a healing activity directed to the whole person in a whole community. Perhaps a chair of 'Health and Theology' might lead to doctoral theses on a wider variety of subjects like 'Surgery and Atonement' or 'Empirical Investigations of Orthodox Medical Healing and the Prophetic Tradition'. There are many signs that the USA, which has the resources to produce a theology of healing which will, in the name of Christ, challenge as well as comfort the practice of medicine all over the world, is turning towards this task. The task is urgent. So hurry up please!

NOTES

1. T. Oden, *Kerygma and Counseling*, Westminster Press, Philadelphia 1966; *Contemporary Theology and Psychotherapy*, Westminster 1968
2. D. Browning, *Atonement and Psychotherapy*, Westminster 1966

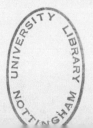